BRAIN
MAINTENANCE

How to Prevent Stroke
&
Delay Dementia

By Kathleen W. Wilson, M.D.

Whiskey Hollow Press
P.O. Box 13752, New Orleans, LA 70185-3752
(866) 329-5710 • (504) 861-2188 • fax (504) 861-1657
www.boomermedicine.com

Although the author and publisher have made every effort to ensure the accurate and completeness of information contained in this book, we assume no responsibility for errors, inaccuracies, omissions, or any inconsistency herein. Any slight of people, places, or organizations is unintentional.

Edited by Joy Parker and Kathleen W. Wilson, MD
Library of Congress Catalog Card Number: 2004103323
ISBN: 0-9742976-4-X
616.81

ATTENTION CORPORATIONS, UNIVERSITIES, COLLEGES,
AND PROFESSIONAL ORGANIZATIONS:
Quantity discounts are available in bulk purchases of this book for educational, gift purposes, as premiums for increasing magazine subscription or renewals. Special books or book excerpts can also be created to fit specific needs. For information, please contact Whiskey Hollow Press, P.O. Box 13752, New Orleans, LA 70185-3752. (866) 329-5710 (504) 861-2188/(504) 861-1657 fax. www.boomermedicine.com.

Acknowledgements

I was able to write this with the help of my partners at Ochsner Clinic Foundation. Drs. Robert Felberg and Kevin McKinley of Ochsner Clinic Neurology helped me with this cutting edge information. Drs. Susan Vaught and Susan Vogel helped me with the tests for dementia. Dr. Ken Miller, Neuroradiologist, spent time and effort to teach me the intricacies of CAT scans and MRI's of the brain and Dr. O. Nachar of Nuclear Medicine helped me with PET and SPECT scans. Thanks to Dr. Laura Serpa, Dr. Lillian Lesser, Merri Ferrell, Robert Bach, and Dr. Don Rugg for reading the manuscript as it evolved and giving me feedback. Thanks to Dr. John Phipps who helped me write about the effects of alcoholism on the brain. I appreciate the well wishes of good luck from Drs. Edelman, Snowdon, and Vaillant.

A special thanks to my husband, Dr. Mike Wilson for his wit, support, editing, conceiving the book cover, and making this important information more readable.

I will always hold the doctors at Mayo Clinic who taught me the art and science of medicine, in highest esteem. In particular, the Mayo psychiatrists and neurologists were superb teachers and I could never have understood these concepts, or written this book without their teaching. As a Mayo Clinic trained doctor, I was positioned to help many patients through the years. Mayo's training was second to none.

I thank Joy Parker for editing this book. Thanks to Rebecca O'Meara for her innovative and savvy business, promotion and marketing ideas and to Stephanie Robison of Upside Design for her witty cover and graphic design of the book.

Disclaimer

Everything I wrote I currently believe to be true about brain preservation and this is how I practice medicine. But in medicine, we are always questioning what we believe, so some of the information could become outdated as research advances the state of medical knowledge.

Although this information is generally helpful, I am not prescribing what any individual should do. He or she must consult with his or her own doctor because everyone's situation is different. The contents of the book are my professional opinion and I am not speaking for other doctors including those who have shared their viewpoints and helped me with the book, or written their own book. I do not intend this book as a standard of care reference.

The persons in the stories are disguised and personal details are changed so there is no way that anyone can recognize himself, except for the one instance where a generous patient said to me, "If I can help someone else with my story, please tell it."

I wade into the controversies of the Women's Health Initiative studies on hormone replacement therapy. Although my opinion differs from the study's authors and some of the other writers who have interpreted the WHI results for the public, I intend no disrespect and am in no way discrediting the effort of the WHI research team. I am only stating my opinion.

Brain Maintenance:
How to Prevent Stroke & Delay Dementia

Table of Contents

Introduction

As we mature, we are often responsible for weighty decisions affecting others, so we are duty bound to protect our brain cells. If our reasoning is flawed by brain disease, the outcome may be disastrous. You may have seen *Sum of All Fears*, the movie based on Tom Clancy's book. Just as senior government leaders are trying to decide whether to launch a nuclear weapon and decimate 25 million people, one of the men has a heart attack. When someone's cardiovascular system collapses, it's a sure thing that he is not getting enough oxygen to his brain to make a decision like this.

We hear of decisions that, to put it mildly, often seem like bad choices. These stories make us shake our heads and wonder "Who made that call?!" For example, why did senior officials (according to inferences in the media) tell younger FBI agents to stop following those Al Queda guys – and withdraw the resources to do so a few weeks before 9/11? Could impaired mental function due to brain disease seen with aging be part of the answer? Another area where puzzling mistakes are often made is the NASA program. NASA's space shuttle disasters have been euphemistically referred to as "a problem with NASA culture." But is it possible that the upper echelon of management and safety control was not as focused as it should have been on some of the complexities and dangers of the manned space flights they orchestrated?

Can we be confident that the crucial decision makers in our country are doing everything known to science to preserve the edge and integrity of their mental processes? Or do these men and women suffer from the same declining mental function that many ordinary citizens experience as they age?
In other words, not everyone gets wiser as they get older.

Why I Wrote This Book...
So You Could Worry Less

This book is for people with normal mental function. Unfortunately, it cannot help those who already have dementia. By then, it is too late.

Now for the good news: Dementia is not a normal part of aging and can be prevented in many cases. Most people do not know that. Even if they do suspect that there are things they can do to help themselves stay sharp, they probably don't have the latest medical information about what those things are.

The world can cause us many anxieties. Some we can do nothing about. I feel badly about migrant farm workers who are exploited, children in my own community who do not have the same opportunities I had, hurricanes, and deadly viruses that spread around the world with globalization. Unfortunately, I have little or no influence on these events.

Yet, based on research findings from the last few years, I know that I can influence my future mental function. Whether or not I maintain my mental function into my senior years is largely within my control.

So far, dementia is not very treatable once it is well established. The pharmaceutical industry is working hard to find something that prevents the brain lesions of Alzheimer's, but once the damage is done, brain tissue does not repair itself. So the time to think about maintaining your brain is now, while you still can.

What This Book Will Tell You

Risk factors fall into two categories: the ones that you inherit and the ones that you can avoid or change. Even if you have inherited a genetic tendency to develop a disease, there are still things that you can do to steer clear of it, if you start early enough. This book gives you the tools to prevent adding more brain damage to the impairment that might occur with age, and outlines the choices you must make now. It is the additive effects of multiple small brain injuries superimposed on varying degrees of Alzheimer's changes in the aging brain that cause dementia, that final common pathway of brain failure.

How the Book Is Organized

The first third of this book presents the latest theories about the causes of dementia, as well as leading-edge information on normal brain development. This landmark research includes:

• An analysis of The Nun Study, a breakthrough study on dementia conducted

by Dr. David Snowdon and published in his book *Aging with Grace*
- An examination of Nobel Prize winner Dr. Gerald M. Edelman's theories of brain function, development and adaptable brain tracts
- A discussion of the Grant Study by Harvard psychiatrist Dr. George Vaillant, which explored factors that lead to happiness, health and clear mental function later in life, and factors that leave some people bereft and alone
- I will tell you what CAT scans, PET scans and MRI's of the brain show us, and explain the thinking behind tests of brain function for adults.
- The second part of the book goes into detail about Alzheimer's disease, probably the single most feared degenerative illness of the brain.
- The third part of the book discusses the effects of stroke (a.k.a., loss of blood flow to parts of the brain, resulting in brain cell death).

Please notice that the causes and treatment of dementia, stroke and hypertension overlap. Most importantly, understand that the factors that lead to stroke and damage from hypertension are under your control.

About the Author

I began practicing medicine full-time when I finished medical school in 1975. Since 1993, I have been an internal (adult) medicine doctor at the internationally respected Ochsner Clinic Foundation in New Orleans. Ochsner Clinic Foundation is a group practice of over four hundred staff physicians and two hundred and fifty resident physicians in training. We have doctors in all specialties and subspecialties practicing in one large clinic, and thirty smaller neighborhood clinics, resulting in over a million patient visits annually. Our facilities include a six hundred-bed hospital, operating rooms, an emergency room, critical care units, laboratories and radiology.

As an internist, I see over four thousand patients a year, ages eighteen to one hundred. My patients come from all walks of life and are as racially diverse as this magical port city of New Orleans. African-Americans, Vietnamese, Hispanics, Caucasians of all ethnic mixtures, Cajuns (French-Canadians who moved to Louisiana over two hundred years ago), New Orleanians from old families, Yankees (a lot of us live in New Orleans and love our city), and Muslim and Hindu patients are all under my care. I write about what I have learned from my Mayo Clinic training, my patients, colleagues, and reading medical journals. Ochsner Clinic Foundation's neurologists and psychiatrists helped me to refine the concepts in this book.

When I entered medical school in 1971 at the University of Iowa, we were taught what we needed to become good doctors who take excellent care of our patients. In 1975 I went to Mayo Clinic for my three-year internal medicine residency and two-year gastroenterology fellowship. I cannot imagine any better medical training than what I received from the doctors at Mayo Clinic. The seven and one half months I was assigned to Mayo's neurology and psychiatry services gave me a solid background for following the science of brain function.

After five years of private practice in Iowa, from 1985 to 1993, I was on active duty in the Air Force as Chief of Executive Medicine and doctor to the active duty and retired general officers and their wives. There I had the opportunity to meet intelligent, talented individuals, people who made history. I observed these patients in the fourth, fifth, sixth, seventh and eighth decade of their lives, and came to understand what kept them healthy and mentally sharp. I witnessed the effects of good lifestyles and bad ones, and learned to identify where potential trouble lurked. That is when I began thinking about medicine differently, not just as the practice of treating a disease that was presenting itself at any given moment, but as a lifelong process, the goal of which is to shepherd people to good health.

Before We Begin, Some Useful Definitions

Because doctors, patients and families use the words **Alzheimer's disease, dementia,** and **stroke** loosely, I need to begin by defining these terms so that this book is clear and understandable.

Unless a person has died and his or her brain has been examined under the microscope, you can only say someone has probable Alzheimer's. The brains of Alzheimer's patients show characteristic sticky microscopic plaques of amyloid, degenerated proteins, and tangles that once were effective paths of communication among brain cells. They also show a marked loss of brain cells.

In recent years, however, PET scans of the brain have become so specific that the results correlate closely with the autopsy findings of Alzheimer's. Thus, I will use the term Alzheimer's, when I am talking about the physical damage – the cellular changes of the disease or the PET scan findings.

Otherwise, I will use the term dementia. Dementia refers not to what one sees physically in the brain, but what one sees clinically in the patient's behavior. It literally means "lost mind," that sorry state we so fret about when we see it in our older relatives and extrapolate that we must be sitting ducks, next in line for this fate worse than death. Though the terms have been used so often as to become almost interchangeable, there is one clear distinction between them. Many causes and conditions can lead to the loss of function that we label as dementia, and Alzheimer's is just one of them.

Having a stroke means that your brain cells have died because blocked blood vessels cannot supply proper amounts of oxygen and nutrients to them. Stroke and Alzheimer's probably cause dementia synergistically. This is one of the key points of this book.

Charlie Worries about His Mental Function

Charlie, a 53-year-old man, is overloaded. At work, he does the job of three people. When two coworkers were laid off, he had to take over for them without complaining or he would have been next in line for the pink slip. Since then, his work week has ballooned to over 50 hours.

Charlie has other obligations besides work. When he gets home, he is responsible for household tasks because his wife works outside the home as well. He has a teenager who is going through a rough phase and acting out, so he also has to cope with emotional upheavals in the family.

His older parents live in town and expect him to visit them once a week. In spite of the fact that he complies with their wishes, they complain that they never see him. He is troubled during these visits because his father, formerly mentally sharp, often repeats his stories, forgets what he is saying in conversation, and gets irritable about nothing. Charlie's mother watches over his father as though she is afraid of what he is going to say or do next.

When Charlie reached fifty, strange things started happening to his mind. He had always relied on his intellect and wit to get him through the most difficult situations with grace. He went to a party a few months ago, saw an old friend from high school, his best buddy back then, and couldn't think of the guy's name. He could have kept that to himself, but someone else walked up and expected Charlie to introduce them. Though he stumbled through the introduction, it was a jarring experience.

When he gave a presentation at work a few weeks ago, in the middle of a sentence, he forgot the word he meant to say. He just stammered, "You know, I mean…" and felt foolish. He remembered the word thirty minutes later, but the audience had left the room by then and there was no one to whom he could say that his memory hadn't had a breakdown. These days it just takes him a little longer.

Sometimes he finds himself getting overly upset and not being able to calm down for awhile. He used to be able to laugh things off more quickly. Now he finds himself looking forward to his two nightly martinis to relieve his stress.

Charlie hasn't been to a doctor for ten years. He doesn't want to take the time off to get a thorough physical because he's heard that navigating the medical system is more difficult than getting through airline security these days. He doesn't want to wait an hour in a waiting room; it would make him too angry. He is also afraid of what the doctor will tell him, and is convinced that he probably wouldn't want to take pills, even if the doctor said he needed medicine for things such as high cholesterol or hypertension.

Nevertheless, there is that nagging question in the back of Charlie's mind. What if his father is getting Alzheimer's disease? And what if his own strange lapses mean he is in the early stages of this dreadful illness?

What if Charlie's doctor could offer him a way to prevent dementia? The truth is, he or she can.

Normal Brain
Development

Normal Brain Changes with Age

The Simple Version

The human brain matures through late middle age, both intellectually and emotionally. New connections between brain cells are continually being made, which can result in better integration and more mental complexity. You can help these positive changes along by interacting with other people, loving your family, learning new things, reading interesting books, and engaging in creative projects. All these abilities are part of the gift of being human and keep the mind active, flexible and sharp.

The Details

To begin, let's define a number of terms that are crucial to understanding how brain cells function.

Brain cells consist of a nerve body, with a long extension, the axon, which carries information to other nerve cells. Synapses are connections between brain cells. Many chemicals called neurotransmitters, such as serotonin, norepinephrine, and dopamine, pass across these synapses, allowing brain cells to communicate with each other. Gray matter is the outer coating of the brain that contains the nerve cells. White matter, the part of the brain that contains all those long brain connections, is found just beneath the gray matter. Myelin is the white sheath that wraps around the extensions of nerve cells (like insulation) and accelerates cell to cell communication. One could say that myelin is as important to the speedy delivery of brain messages as Federal Express is to mail.

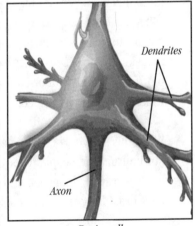

Dendrites

Axon

Brain cell

The weight of the human brain reaches its maximum at age 29, but the sophisticated part of the brain that reasons and feels, the part that one might call "mind" instead of just the physical brain, continues to add myelin for decades. This myelin, which enhances cell to cell communication, reaches its maximum development between the ages of 50 and 60. This means that brain development, and intellectual and emotional complexity continues until ages 50 to 60.

Ben is a successful businessman. When he was in his early 20's, he focused on developing his skills in business and completed an MBA degree. In his late 20's he married, but often took his wife for granted and left the management of the house and his three children, and their social and family relationships to her exclusively. In his 30's, Ben consolidated his success, earning several million dollars as a business entrepreneur. Some referred to him as a visionary. Others called him a workaholic.

When Ben reached age 45, his brother committed suicide. He did not see that tragedy coming but it was a dramatic wake-up call. Suddenly he felt more vulnerable and began to question whether never-ending work was how he wanted to live the rest of his life. When Ben first told his wife that he wanted more time to talk to her about his feelings, she was skeptical of this abrupt change in his personality. Finally, he persuaded her that his desire to spend more time with her and the children and less time in the office was genuine. Other changes soon followed. Ben started calling his parents once a week, initially to make sure they were coping with the shock of his brother's death, but later, just to see how they were. He rearranged his schedule so that he had more time off and followed a lifelong dream to write short stories, a few of which were even published.

While this story is a composite of several of my male patients at midlife, it is not unusual for people to become more sensitive to the feelings of others, their own inner longings, and to reach out for more human connection as their brain becomes more complex.

The Brain is Not a Computer

Let me introduce you to Dr. Gerald M. Edelman's theory of brain development and function. His explanation of how the brain works is the best theory I have read. Dr. Edelman is a Nobel Prize winner and head of the Neurosciences Institute of San Diego. Many years ago he became fascinated by the question of what makes us "mindful." Why are human beings so different from one another, he asked, so emotionally rich and complex? Why are they versatile enough to be able to adapt to situations the brain has never before encountered?

Dr. Edelman discusses all of these ideas and more in his book, *A Universe of Consciousness; How Matter Becomes Imagination*. His first broad stroke is to say that the brain couldn't possibility be a genetically predetermined organ that already has all the nerve cells and connections it needs. That theory would not account for the human ability to learn and remember. Rather, he thinks the brain is physically and chemically designed to be able to adapt to the unknowns we encounter around every corner.

In his theory, there is only a basic structure in place at birth. Before birth, brain cells move around, reproduce, marry up to one another with biologic adhesive, and make many connections to other cells with whom they communicate closely. The genetic structure only gives a general outline for the location and connections of the neurons.

Developmental selection is how Edelman describes what happens after birth. The location and connections of the brain cells stabilize at birth. Then certain groups, what he calls "maps" of brain cells, begin to build basic brain functions when stimulated by a new experience. For example, consider the miracle of vision. As babies we start with basic programming. The retina – brain cells at the back of the eye – receives an image, and then the optic pathways move this image to the back of the brain, which recognizes that we are seeing something. The brain responds by sending the image to a number of other brain centers where it can be identified, interpreted, and put into the context of other things that were previously seen. In this way a whole gallery of images – and their relationships to one another – can be built up.

Developmental selection is clearly different from a computer with its completely engineered circuitry. A computer can only do what it is programmed to do. It cannot grow and adapt to its experiences.

Edelman reasons that a child learns to walk because he comes up against the problem of crossing the room, not just because his brain has grown to the point where he is able to walk. This is an example of how the billions of connections between brain cells and "maps" of brain cells either strengthen or die out during a lifetime of experiences as the brain adapts and develops useful skills. While a child learning to walk is an example of a new connection getting stronger, my college French, which I haven't used since 1970, is an example of a brain tract that has atrophied. It is unlikely that I could bring my old facility with that language back to life in my brain without a lot of review.

On the other hand, my brain tracts that have the ability to process complex patient problems have hypertrophied – grown stronger. For this reason, medicine is much easier to practice than when I was a young doctor just learning about these things. Edelman thinks the brain develops passageways and skills because of life's challenges.

So, from the time a child is born, every thought and stimulus has an impact on these critical neuronal connections that make up the mind. Edelman calls this **experiential selection.** What that process means for us is profound. If our brains are modified by our thoughts, friendships, experiences, relationships, and hardships, then we have the freedom to choose how our brains change with age. A person with mean, narrow-minded parents is free to become kind and giving. An explosive person can learn to manage his anger. We can acquire new interests with age, make new friends, and experience new challenges, all of which are good for maintaining the brain. Edelman's theory also explains why people can become happier as they age. By midlife they have already encountered many of life's obstacles, and their brains have learned to adapt. So things should get easier as they go along.

Edelman believes that a memory is retrieved by nests or "maps" of brain cells relating to one another. Memory does not just sit in one cell waiting to be called up. Rather, subsets of information can combine to form a whole memory. For example, take a concept such as "my Aunt Nettie." That name involves a picture of her, an emotional impression, the meaning of the word aunt, and other associations. Each of these parts of Aunt Nettie resides in different groups "maps" of nerve cells. Stimulation of any one of these groups, e.g., the smell of the fresh baked apple pie she used to make, re-creates the image you have of Aunt Nettie by stimulating all the "maps" related to her.

This theory could also explain how poetry is written, if we think of poetry as the association of many different groups of cells. Complex thoughts come about through the regrouping and re-stimulation of a multitude of nests of connected brain cells. Edelman believes that there is constant circulation in the brain of thoughts, feelings and symbols.

The third part of Edelman's theory is called **re-entry,** which is the reconstruction of skills, memories, and brain function through thousands of parallel connections between sites of brain cells. The more tracts a person creates through learning and experience, the more redundant connections between brain cells he has to call upon later in life. If the destructive changes of Alzheimer's take away some of the connections and nests of brain cells, the collateral routes will prevent dementia. If an older person starts to develop some of the physical brain changes of Alzheimer's, and if that is all that is wrong with his or her brain, then they may be able to activate these parallel pathways and go on thinking and feeling with little deleterious effect. This explains why social interaction and ongoing mental stimulation keep people sharp.

I have an 84-year-old patient, Miss Edna, who is a volunteer at a home for troubled children. She goes to the home four days a week and stays six hours at a time. I know that she has arthritis and is on several medicines for her blood pressure and her heart condition, but whenever I ask how she is, she tells me that she feels wonderful. One day I asked her, "Why do you work so hard at this volunteer job? Doesn't being around those kids tire you?"

"Not at all," she said. "Those children need me. There is nothing better I could be doing with my time. I don't want recognition and I'm not doing this so my friends think I'm a good person. I am doing this because it is the right thing and because I love it. I know I can make a difference in these kids' lives." And she is right. She has helped several troubled children negotiate the rough waters of their teenage years and encouraged a few of them to go on to college. There is no doubt that what she is doing is difficult, but it also develops her intellect and her emotional centers, and keeps her focused on the needs of others. I see no signs of dementia in her.

Another 70-year-old male patient of mine named Robert had a religious calling later in life through which he connected with others. Robert helped me out in a tough situation seven years ago. One of my patients, a very old woman, had to undergo treacherous surgery to correct a painful, displaced metal replacement hip ball and socket. This woman's condition was so dire she sometimes screamed with pain and the problem could only be corrected by surgery. Unfortunately I felt certain that with all her underlying medical problems she would probably die during or immediately following the operation. She lived alone and was friendless in a small country town, except for a retarded neighbor boy who looked in on her. Our backs were to the wall, trying to figure out how to get her through the surgery.

When a few of the people who worked with us at Ochsner felt that a prayer vigil would help this woman, we called Robert for help. He got together all the people in his group to pray for this poor old woman. Amazingly, she made it through the surgery with a beautiful post-op result, no residual pain after she healed, and no complications. When I thanked Robert for his help later that year, he quietly told me that he and his friends had visited the old woman while she was in the hospital to give her comfort and support. Robert is not going to get dementia. His sense of compassion – and his brain – are too highly developed.

Terry is in a much different situation. She took an early retirement, lives alone, does nothing more than watch television most days and never exercises. When I ask Terry how she feels, she says "I'm falling apart." Then she goes on to enumerate five to ten physical complaints. It is too early to judge what the effect of her isolated lifestyle and poor health habits will be on her future mentation, but I wouldn't be willing to place any bets on her mental clarity into her 70's and her 80's. If I had to hedge my bets, I'd place them on the brain health of the 84-year-old Miss Edna I told you about earlier.

Another sad case is a 48-year-old woman patient, Jane, who works at a job she hates, has had at least two divorces, smokes, and feels like a victim. Anti-depressants haven't helped her at all, although several psychiatrists have tried to do what they could for her. I have managed to get Jane's blood pressure under control, but I can't foresee excellent brain function for her later in life. From what we understand about how to avoid dementia, Jane's lifestyle is all wrong.

The Nun Study

The Simple Version

Head trauma, stroke and folic acid deficiency predispose patients to dementia who have the brain changes caused by Alzheimer's. Alzheimer's disease may begin before age 20 and progress in some people for a lifetime, but the dementia is not recognized until later in life.

The Details

The Nun Study by epidemiologist Dr. David Snowdon represents some of the finest breakthrough work on dementia that has been published over the last few years. I highly recommend his book, *Aging with Grace,* which tells the story of this study.

Snowdon studied 678 retired Catholic sisters, aged 75 to 102, who were living in retirement convents. He chose this group because of the uniformity of their diet, medical care and lifestyle. They did not smoke and none took estrogen after menopause. Snowdon carefully tested their mental functions from 1991 until they died—the study is ongoing in those nuns who are living. The nuns donated their brains to science after death so that autopsies could be performed. This allowed Snowdon to correlate the physical changes of Alzheimer's with the nuns' intellectual abilities during the last years of their lives. Over 800 brain autopsies have been done so far.

As an epidemiologist, Snowdon has been working to understand the multiple root causes of the complex problem of late life dementia so that it can be prevented. The Nun Study sheds an enormous amount of light on what we can do to help ourselves prevent dementia.

Brain Reserve

One of the questions in the study of dementia focuses on what scientists call brain reserve or the redundancy of connections in the brain. Do some people have so much brain reserve that they can still function well even if they do lose some brain cells to the ravages of Alzheimer's or some other dementing disease? Can the brain be "exercised" or built up by maintaining interests and learning? The answer to these questions is "Yes." Snowdon is careful not to say that more intelligent people have a lower risk of dementia. He does make observations about the effect of education, however. The Catholic sisters who had a college degree were more likely to maintain physical and mental vitality late in life, and to be able to take care of themselves without assistance. Therefore, he concluded that education and learning may increase brain reserve.

Brain reserve might also have a genetic component. In other words, from birth some brains may be more resilient and effective than others, more able to adapt to and circumvent damage to brain cells.

Age and Dementia

Aging is the biggest predictor of dementia. Half of those who live into their nineties now suffer from some form of dementia. But there are also people in their nineties who show no signs of dementia. In other words, the brain does not always "wear out" with the passage of time. In the Nun Study, the autopsies showed that about 40 percent of the elderly sisters who died after age 96 had minimal Alzheimer's changes.

How the Nuns' Autobiographies, Written at Age 20, Predicted Dementia Later in Life

Snowdon describes finding an epidemiologist's treasure in the convent's historical room. Many of the records of the sisters' schooling and family histories had been carefully preserved, as well as the nuns' autobiographies written when they entered the religious order at the average age of 22. Snowdon and a psycholinguist analyzed 93 of these autobiographies. Here are their findings and conclusions.

The sisters who had more resilient brains later in life tended to use multi-syllable words in their early autobiographies and had a richer vocabulary. Those who developed dementia later on used simpler, single syllable words. What is most significant, however, is the **density of ideas**, which Snowdon defines as the number of ideas per ten words. Idea density reflects the brain's ability to process language, remember, and integrate thoughts.

Snowdon discovered that the idea density in early adulthood predicted with an 80 percent accuracy which of the nuns would have good mental function and which would get dementia almost five decades later. These differences did not always correlate with the sisters' level of education or the grades they made in high school.

What this may mean is that the mind is like a muscle that needs exercise, including social connection, ongoing learning, and work of some complexity. It is also possible that some people have excess brain capacity and are less likely to become demented later on in life.

On a more ominous note, those essays that contained a low density of ideas may have predicted who would develop Alzheimer's later on because this disease begins before the age of 20 and is only noticeable with aging. Another conclusion that could be drawn is that not thinking imaginatively at a young age may make the brain more susceptible to Alzheimer's changes. Here we have the classic conundrum, "Which came first, the chicken or the egg?"

If readers doubt that Alzheimer's can start early in life, I would like to direct you to the work of Dr. H. Braak. This highly respected neuropathologist reported changes indicative of early Alzheimer's in the brains of deceased 20-year-olds. In nearly one hundred articles in scientific journals, Braak describes the progression of Alzheimer's over 50 years of life, from stage I through stage VI. The earliest plaques and tangles are found near the memory part of the brain. In the late stages Alzheimer's reaches the gray matter, that top covering of the human brain that allows the most intricate intellectual and social functioning.

Using Dr. Braak's classification system of the severity of Alzheimer's in autopsied brains, Snowdon discovered the following:

- 22 percent of the nuns whose autopsied brains had stage I to stage II Alzheimer's, showed signs of dementia prior to death.
- 43 percent of the nuns whose autopsied brains had stage III to stage IV Alzheimer's, showed signs of dementia before death.
- 70 percent of the nuns whose autopsied brains had stage V to stage VI

Alzheimer's, showed signs of dementia before death.

However, some sisters with minor physical brain changes were demented while others with severe changes scored fairly well on their adult IQ tests up until death. This shows that other factors than Alzheimer's changes influence brain function later in life.

The brains of sisters who had significant dementia while alive were shrunken at autopsy. The normal mature female brain weighs between 1100-1800 grams, or two to three pounds. The brains of the Alzheimer's victims had shrunk to less than 1000 grams. The complex grooves in the gray matter of these brains had become smooth with large gaps between the peaks of convoluted brain tissue.

The Gene for Alzheimer's

The amyloid plaques we see in the brains of those with Alzheimer's disease are formed in part via the chemical pathway involved with cholesterol. Apolipoprotein E (APOE) is a genetic marker for a protein carrier of cholesterol that comes in three basic forms, 2, 3 and 4. A person gets one APOE gene from each parent. APOE-4 is the gene that is associated with the plaques and tangles of Alzheimer's. If a person has a single copy of the APOE-4 gene from one of his parents, he has three times the risk of getting the disease in later life. If he receives a copy from both parents, which would mean that he has two APOE-4 genes, his risk is increased eightfold.

In the Nun Study, 20 percent of the sisters had a single copy of the APOE-4 gene and 2.6 percent had two copies. If you have two copies of the APOE-4 gene, it is far less likely that you will be able to prevent dementia within your lifetime.

I asked a non-doctor friend age 50 to read this manuscript. She said, "This raises the question of "How would you know? Are you saying that people should get genetic testing? If someone learns that they have two copies of this gene can you give them some hope?" The answer is that genetic testing is not recommended because knowing you have two copies of APOE-4 is a burden you do not want to bear while life is still normal for you. Doctors may check for two APOE-4 genes when they are trying to make a correct diagnosis in a relatively young person with signs of dementia. Given the limitations of our present treatments, this is the only time that genetic testing for this disease would be useful.

I bring this up here because I want to make the point that there are a few unusual genetic problems that will eventually result in dementia, and the people who have them are blameless. This minority of patients could not have exercised more, eaten more vegetables, or done anything else to prevent their genetic predetermination. These unfortunate patients are treated with drugs that help stabilize memory and more effective drugs are being developed.

Stroke, Head Trauma, and Folic Acid in the Nun Study
There were three other significant elements that seemed to be present in the bodies of the nuns who died with noticeable symptoms of dementia.

Many sisters with diminished mental capacity were found, at autopsy, to show evidence of stroke and atherosclerosis in the blood vessels supplying the brain. Atherosclerosis is a degenerative disease resulting from the build up of plaques consisting of dead cells, lipids, and cholesterol crystals in the artery walls. Snowdon and his colleagues believe these sisters showed signs of dementia because stroke prevents brain cells from communicating with each other.

Head trauma also raised the risk of dementia. The pathologist could see the scars from the old accidents when the brains were examined after death.

Lastly, there was a direct correlation between the level of folic acid present in the blood and brain function. When the folic acid level was high, the sisters were sharper. Folic acid lowers the level of homocysteine. High levels of homocysteine may cause stroke as well as toxicity to brain cells.

In closing, please let me reiterate the factors in the Nun Study found to cause dementia in the nuns. The nuns who lacked complexity of thought early in life were more likely to have dementia in old age. Those with stroke were much more likely to have dementia if they also had changes of Alzheimer's at autopsy. And the nuns with higher folic acid levels (and thus lower homocysteine) were sharper. Brain trauma also contributed to dementia.

Therefore the Nun Study tells us that we must prevent stroke (and I will tell you how), avoid head trauma, take folic acid, and try to be optimistic and engaged in life if we want to prevent or delay dementia.

The Grant Study and
Dr. George E. Vaillant's Work

The Simple Version

Dr. George Vaillant's life's work as an eminent psychiatrist and researcher at Harvard focused on what allows people to age successfully and enjoy life up until the end. He found that the joy of living leads to successful aging. Gratitude, forgiveness, and loving are important to happiness later in life. Is happiness a factor in not developing dementia? It's hard to say, but in my experience as a physician, generous-hearted people who have strong connections with others have less apparent trouble with brain function, or perhaps they have less trouble with life and its vicissitudes. For example, Vaillant points out that having a good marriage at age 50 predicts successful aging (in the group of men he studied), whereas alcohol abuse, which leads a person into an isolated lifestyle, inevitably causes mental and physical decline, loneliness, and early death.

Perhaps the larger question posed by Vaillant's work is this: What do you want your brain to be able to do later in life? Perhaps the proof of a well-maintained brain is not so much still being able to do calculus, but having the love of your family, making helpful contributions to others, and having a sense of well-being.

The Details

Drs. Vaillant and Edelman are in agreement, from the perspective of a psychiatrist and a neurology researcher, respectively, that the human brain continues to mature into middle age. Our genetic makeup is set from conception, but encoded in our genes is the brain's ability to adapt and change.

Of what value is a long life with an efficiently functioning brain if a person has not learned the skills that create happiness? That is the question that Harvard psychiatrist George E. Vaillant answered in his book, *Aging Well*. For a minimum of 50 years, from early adulthood on, the lives of two groups of men and one group of women were studied to see which factors and lifestyles lead to happiness and health later in life, and which choices leave some people bereft and alone.

The first group, called the Grant Study, was comprised of 268 socially advantaged, well-adjusted Harvard sophomores followed for sixty years by Dr. Vaillant and his predecessors directing the study. Every two years, these individuals completed questionnaires and underwent psychological interviews, enabling researchers to track key events of their lives.

The second group, the Glueck Study, was comprised of 456 disadvantaged, white inner city men born about 1930, mainly of Irish and Italian descent, whose parents were often recent immigrants to America. Vaillant was able to find and interview most of them once while they were in their 60's.

The third group, the Terman Study, followed 90 middle-class, white women from their early school years in California. These women, most of whom were born about 1910, were selected for the study because they were intellectually gifted. Although the Terman Study had been disbanded years before, Vaillant located and interviewed 40 of these women one time who were still alive.

Mature Defenses

Vaillant found that a person's basic unconscious ego defenses against life's big and small miseries have a lot to do with their happiness as they age. These defenses determine the way people bounce back, and unload something bad while minimizing anxiety.

The mature defenses are humor, sublimation (taking the energy from a blocked desire or sadness and turning it into a positive endeavor), altruism (giving selflessly to others), and suppression (plain old stoicism). People who use mature ego defenses are generally easier to get along with.

Roy was a master of humor. When I had to tell him one kidney wasn't working properly, and that his arthritis would soon require surgery, Roy just smiled and said, "My father gave me two words of advice. 'Don't weaken.'"

By sublimation, Vaillant means the manner in which some people can deal with socially unacceptable impulses, feelings, and ideas in socially acceptable ways. Sublimation is a mature defense mechanism because it channels feelings and desires that are socially out of bounds, into behaviors that are socially tolerable or appropriate.

Here is an example of sublimation. Mr. Allen is bedeviled by desire for his younger partner's wife, Jackie. He knows that if he pursues that desire, it could destroy the happiness of Jackie and her young family, he could lose his long-term marriage, and his senior law partners may condemn him. Mr. Allen wisely decides to keep the thoughts of Jackie's attractiveness to himself. Instead Mr. Allen mentors his younger partner, Jackie's husband, teaching him the nuances of the law and this particular firm. Mr. Allen respectfully declines the younger family's invitation to dinner.

David, another patient, is an altruist. He has suffered for years with the worst rheumatoid arthritis I have ever seen. I had never seen David out of a wheelchair. In spite of his pain, he has befriended an 88-year-old woman with dementia, carefully makes sure she takes her medicine properly, and accompanies her to her doctors' appointments.

Ed is a patient who exemplifies stoicism. Since he has pulmonary fibrosis, and scar tissue in his lungs, he is often short of breath and unable to stop coughing. When Ed went to a lung specialist and was told that this is not a treatable disease, he said he didn't want to talk about the problem because there was nothing he could do about it anyway. I watched him go on about his life with as much gusto as he could manage. Ed continues to travel with a friend, visiting historical places and bluegrass festivals. His courage strengthens all who know him.

Immature Defenses

The immature defenses that alienate people are projection (blaming something bad about yourself on someone else), and passive aggression (indirectly expressing hostility from behind a façade of compliance).

To illustrate projection, let's say that Lila doesn't like her boss, but rather than acknowledge that, Lila says "The boss doesn't like me." Lila disowns her own negative feeling by giving it to someone else.

Passive aggression is another alienating immature defense. I saw an example of passive aggression in the grocery store a few months ago. This store never has enough people working in the cold cut section so there is always a long line of waiting shoppers. A worker was slowly, precisely slicing cold turkey and cheese, slowly and carefully wrapping it, and then holding it just out of the customer's reach while asking if there was anything else they wanted and suggesting other meats and cheeses that she thought were good. Meanwhile the rest of the people in line were becoming more impatient and exasperated. That employee was acting out her hostility while maintaining a face of sweetness and customer service.

On the farthest end of the negative spectrum are a group of people who are alone because no one seems to care about them. These individuals are almost always divorced or single and have alienated every significant person in their lives. Even medical personnel find it difficult to like them or to feel much sympathy for them although these individuals make frequent appointments because they have so little human contact outside the paid doctor-patient relationship. These unfortunate people often have personality disorders, based on a predominance of immature, offensive ego defenses.

In most cases, Vaillant found that as people age, their defense mechanisms mature and they generally become nicer people. He also discovered that personality growth can be blocked by alcoholism and depression.

Alcoholism

Alcoholism stops the growth of personality and separates the alcoholic from loved ones so that soon he or she is only associating with other alcoholics. Alcohol literally causes brain damage, not just to the balance and memory portions of the brain, but also to the complex emotional centers.

Here are two contrasting stories of the fates of two of my alcoholic patients. These stories are longer than the others in this book because this problem is more complicated, physically, mentally, socially, and spiritually. So bear with me.

The first patient I want you to meet is Jim. Jim spent twenty years as an officer in the Air Force, then retired as a major. He was having gastrointestinal problems when we first met, which were probably either caused or aggravated by his habit of drinking beer all day, nearly every day. His second wife had given up and departed, after trying to deal with him for nearly ten years following his retirement.

Jim was intoxicated by midday, fell asleep on the couch in the afternoon, and then rose to start drinking again most evenings with cronies in a shabby local saloon. He had been retired from the service at the young age of fifty, but had never succeeded with a second career. He tried selling used cars at a nearby dealership, but found that the task of speaking with strangers who came to the lot was more than he could handle easily, so he drank more. He never sold a car, left by mutual agreement after six weeks, and resumed his habits at the local pubs, now beginning earlier in the day.

Things were going downhill for Jim when we met. He had become involved in a minor slugfest at the bar and had gotten the worst of it. Even though the three men involved had done little damage, the police had jailed all of them and the manager wanted Jim to stay away from his bar.

A few days later, Jim was picked up driving while intoxicated en route (to, not from) an alternate watering hole. The offense list grew longer when he "told off" the arresting officer and threatened him. After the judge fined him, the lawyer's fees took what was left of his meager savings.

By this time Jim had alienated almost everyone around him. Becky, his daughter, had moved to California with her new husband and seldom telephoned, even though she was pregnant with Jim's first grandchild. The neighbors avoided him and made little attempt to disguise their low regard.

I easily diagnosed Jim's primary problem by his bloodshot eyes, trembling hands, hypertension, and the smell of stale beer that rose from his body and clothes. His attitude was sullen and he seemed to expect bad news. After a short while, however, he began to trust me a little. He was able to tell me some of his story and to confirm my diagnosis, alcoholism.

I recommended strongly that he stop drinking entirely, not just "cut down." I suggested that he attend some meetings of Alcoholics Anonymous, but he seemed to resist the idea of getting help from others. He said that he was "not that bad yet," and that he would be able to "cut down" his drinking on his own. I doubted his ability to stop drinking without help, but it was his choice. His digestive problems improved a little, but three or four visits later it was obvious that he was drinking daily again.

Jim never returned to the clinic. Three years later he died. Alone in a rented apartment, he had choked on his vomitus and simultaneously bled out from ruptured varices (blood vessels of the esophagus). He had expired several days earlier, but no one had noticed. Finally, neighbors, who regarded him as "a derelict," noticed that his truck was mis-parked, and eventually forced the door to find him dead. He died at sixty-three, a young age for a man who was "not that bad yet."

Colonel John, another patient of mine who suffered from alcoholism, coped with this disease in a completely different way and experienced a completely different outcome. In fact, he has come to be one of my best friends and most trusted advisors.

I first met John when he came in for his annual physical. He was fifty-eight years old, but looked younger. At the time, he had been retired from the Air Force for six years. Five years earlier, with great difficulty, he had given up serious drinking.

His history, medical and otherwise, intrigued me. John's mother was an alcoholic who literally drank herself to death while her only son was in his teens. John's father was a heavy drinker too, but lived longer. John was devoted to the Air Force and flew in Korea and Vietnam. Once he came back from the wars, he began to travel down the alcoholic path clearly blazed by his parents. His drinking progressed relentlessly. By the time he retired from the Air Force, his daily routine, as he describes it, was divided into three more or less equal parts – (1) work, (2) drunk, and (3) something between sleep and an alcoholic coma – same routine most days.

When his wife finally left him, he vowed to quit drinking in hopes that she might forgive him and return. Displaying rare willpower, he went "cold turkey" and sobered up at home – without medical assistance. He suffered severe withdrawal symptoms, convulsions and an unusual neurological complication called Wernicke's syndrome – which included brain damage leading to temporary paralysis of one side of his body. Frightened, he accepted neurological treatment and shortly entered a military residential twenty-eight day alcohol rehabilitation program. Fortunately he was able to recover. In my many years of practice, I have seen very few people who developed such severe withdrawal symptoms recover from them so well.

John's rehab led him to Alcoholics Anonymous, a twelve step prescription now followed by more than two million Americans, and AA led him to an entirely new life he had never imagined. After a year or so, he began to devote himself to helping other alcoholics recover, an activity that had the added advantage of keeping himself sober. "I knew I would surely lie to myself and go back to the bottle unless I did something different," John told me. Currently, he attends four to seven AA meetings a week, and has "sponsored" (helped to recovery) dozens of men. Sober, John is a born leader and now heads the county Alcohol Rehabilitation Center, serving on various committees that address alcohol and drug problems.

John's marriage could not be repaired, but he found a soul mate at an AA group meeting three years after his divorce, and he and his new wife have now been happily married for close to twenty years. There is a gleam of joy in their eyes that would never suggest their shared history as alcoholics. Even though they are now near seventy, they still devote hours every day to helping alcoholics recover.

Even though these two alcoholic patients come from similar career and socio-economic backgrounds, what a difference there is between the outcomes of their two stories! While there are many variables in their lives, the most important is the commitment to recovery. John's recovery has lasted through the years, while poor Jim made only a weak gesture to overcome his life's most important problem.

If you know that you have a serious drinking problem, I can't urge you strongly enough to get help without delay. Your whole life will depend on getting and keeping recovery from this awful malady.

Depression and Dementia

Depression prevents the positive interactions that help to develop and maintain a brain as it ages, and it decreases concentration and the ability to learn new things.

Jacqueline has been depressed all her life. She is married and relies heavily on her husband. Whenever she sees me, she is focused on her bowels, or her depression, or her fatigue, or whatever misery it is that day. When Jacqueline had knee arthritis, she underwent knee surgery but was too depressed to do her part of the rehabilitation by following the instructions of the physical therapist. Therefore she has stiff total knee implants that function poorly and is in a wheelchair whenever I see her. She has been to many psychiatrists over the years, taken numerous anti-depressants, complained of side-effects to all, and no matter what anyone did for her, she never seemed to evolve beyond her depression. Although I have been her doctor for a number of years, Jacqueline has never thanked me for taking her many calls, addressing her more than average number of medical complaints, or continuing to be there for her. I have the feeling she does not see me as a person, just one of those other faceless doctors whose job it is to accompany her on her life's journey. As she ages, Jacqueline is more forgetful and fretful. No one has ever expected much of her, so her mental and physical disabilities are accommodated by her family. It is no surprise to me that this patient is becoming demented because she has always had such an inefficient brain.

I knew a man named Harold who regularly accompanied his wife when she came to see me. He was always quarrelsome and unpleasant, and when his wife was alone with me, she told me that he blew up around the house and never had a good day. Within three years, Harold had lost his memory and had dementia.

The basic question is this: Does the negative personality mean that the person's brain is not functioning as well as the brains of others who are more optimistic and better adapted? Or does dementia cause people to be less inhibited, rude and irritable, and not bother to be polite before they lose the rest of their brain function?

Childhood, Marriage, and Education

Vaillant discovered that an unhappy childhood was a less important indicator of how happy a person would be by midlife than a person's attitude and social relationships.

I have a 50-year-old patient, Steven, who grew up with authoritarian parents who constantly restricted his life with arbitrary rules and regulations. He grew up chafing at authority and with a deeply felt disrespect for people in positions of power. Rather than choosing a life trajectory of revolt against authority figures, the man decided to become an independent entrepreneur. He puts himself into the position of authority and creates around him a work environment in which his employees are encouraged to question the status quo and are rewarded for thinking "outside the box."

Both a long happy marriage and successful navigation of old age depend on developing tolerance, maturity, commitment, and the ability to laugh. It seems to me that Vaillant's claim about advantages of a long marriage may apply primarily to men, since many of the women I meet in my practice are lovely, accomplished and nice people whom one would think should be married. However, due to the scarcity of available men past a certain age, they are single. While these women may not be single by choice, they make the most of their situation and live fulfilled lives.

The last item on Vaillant's list of adult milestones was the importance of education. He found that the more years of education a person has, the more likely he or she is to live long and happily. Vaillant speculates that those who are highly educated can take the long view, believing that they have some control over their lives and that they will be able to take care of themselves. He is careful to differentiate between intelligence and schooling. Having a higher IQ or coming from a family with a high social status does not seem to matter as much as the basic fact of having more education. An individual who is brilliant and does nothing with his gifts, or who comes from a rich family, but never does anything with his life will be less likely to be happy in old age than a person who uses whatever resources and intelligence he was born with to get an education and go forward with his life.

Off-Target Verbosity:
A Speech Style that Alienates Others

Off-target verbosity refers to talking too much, not listening, and drifting from topic to topic. More common with aging, it is attributed to loss of the brain's ability to inhibit a person from saying everything he thinks. It is worsened by stress, such as a family get-together. People with this problem tend to show little interest in their conversational partners but just blabber away about themselves. I have no doubt you know exactly what I am talking about, and understand why this characteristic turns people away. So watch out for it, and work on being a good listener.

I can still recall a painful social occasion that my husband Mike and I attended. Close friends, the Smith's, whose company we had always enjoyed, were hosting his mother from out of town. She was a recently remarried widow.

The Smith's invited us to come to dinner with them. For hours, the stepfather went on and on, discussing everything he had ever read, seen, thought, or done. No one else got a word in edgewise the whole evening. I cannot tell you how boring this man was but you can imagine that anyone with a choice in the matter would only endure this kind of evening once.

Summary of Dr. Vaillant's Conclusions:

Dr. Vaillant made four observations about what factors or attitudes helped a person to build and maintain happiness in their lives as they aged.

- It is the good people you meet, not the bad things that happen, that result in happiness later on.
- Loving, expressing gratitude, and forgiving lead to successful aging.
- Retirement is enjoyable if a person continues to create and learns how to play.
- If you think you are in good health that is more important to your well-being than your actual health problems.

Other Qualities That Result in Healthy Aging
- A stable marriage
- Exercise
- Maintaining normal weight
- Mature ego defense mechanisms (humor, altruism, stoicism, sublimation)
- Non-smoking
- No alcohol abuse
- More years of education
- Allowing give and take in your conversations with others

Those Qualities That Result in Unhealthy, Unhappy Aging
- Smoking and drinking alcohol to excess
- A bad marriage
- Immature ego defenses, resentments, and paranoia
- Depression
- Disease
- Off-target verbosity

CAT Scans and MRI's, PET and SPECT Scans

The Simple Version

The brain shrinks in someone with Alzheimer's disease. The metabolism in key brain areas shuts down. Brain imaging can pinpoint some of these problems.

The Details

Before the invention of CAT scans, MRIs, PET and SPECT scans, doctors had little idea what was going wrong in the brain. Research in neurology entered the modern age with current brain imaging techniques.

Why should an imaging study be done on the brain of a patient who develops a mental change? I recall a case long ago that proves you cannot assume what is wrong with someone's brain without a scan. This story was told to me by a widower who shared this about his deceased wife, Rita. Shortly after he married her, Rita changed personality, became horribly abusive to him and his children, and did not function as a wife or mother, although she could talk, walk and eat. Then Rita died in her 50's. This was before we had CAT scans or MRI's. The cause of death was unknown, so the coroner performed an autopsy. Rita had a large brain tumor that had obviously been growing for years and eventually killed her.

What a difference it might have made to Rita's family and her memory if they had known about the brain tumor while she was alive. However, this kind of condition was hard to diagnose in the early 60's when brain imaging was nearly impossible.

CAT Scans

A CAT (computerized axial tomography) scan uses x-rays to map densities of brain tissue. Various areas of the brain, normal brain tissue, and injured brain tissue all transmit x-rays differently. CAT scans are especially helpful for seeing brain hemorrhage, injuries, and abscesses. Most tumors can also be seen by CAT scan. The best use of a CAT scan in a patient with dementia is to rule out the possibility of unexpected causes of the mental changes. About 5 percent of patients with dementia have an unexpected CAT scan or MRI finding such as a brain tumor or a condition called normal pressure hydrocephalus in which the fluid flow around the brain is blocked. Both of these conditions are referred to the neurosurgeon because he or she may be able to correct them with brain surgery.

Our most experienced neuroradiologist at Ochsner told me this story. He had a friendly neighbor, Albert, a retired man, who worked in his garden almost daily, walked in the evening with his wife, and often stopped for a chat. Then, over a six month period, Albert became demented, could barely stand up, was incontinent (lost urine unknowingly) and stopped all his previous activity. Albert was fortunate because the Ochsner neuroradiologist had carefully observed all of these changes and suspected that the older man had one of the rare forms of treatable dementia.

When a CAT scan was done, it confirmed normopressure hydrocephalus, a build up of spinal fluid in the brain when it does not drain properly, putting pressure on the brain. The classic triad of symptoms is dementia, inability to walk, and incontinence. After the diagnosis was made, Ochsner's neurosurgeon was able to shunt the fluid and relieve the pressure on the brain. Albert returned to a semblance of his former self. This is an example of why a CAT scan of the brain may be helpful in a person with the diagnosis of dementia.

I recall another older patient of mine, Kenneth. His wife made an appointment for him, telling me that he had not been himself lately. When Kenneth got up on the exam table, he lay crossways, and nearly fell off. The wife did all the talking because he was unable to recall what his symptoms were. We did a CAT scan and found that Kenneth had a chronic subdural hematoma, a blood clot on the outside of his brain that was causing a build-up of pressure. He probably had fallen weeks ago and struck his head

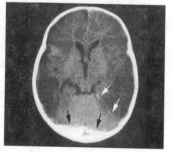

Subdural hematoma

but had not realized it, and the bleeding had been slowly going on all this time. The neurosurgeon drained the blood clot through a burr hole drilled in his skull, and Kenneth returned to his former self, although he was never as sharp as a man his age might be at his best.

When it comes to diagnosing Alzheimer's, a CAT scan is not infallible. While the brain of a patient with Alzheimer's will often look shrunken on a CAT scan, there have been many cases when the brains of patients with dementia look normal. Conversely, a person's brain may appear shrunken on a CAT scan even when the person is not demented.

The Benefits of an MRI

Instead of x-rays, MRI (magnetic resonance imaging) uses a strong magnetic field that measures the response of each hydrogen atom in the body to the magnet. The intensity of the response of the hydrogen atoms in the brain during an MRI depends upon the water content of the brain tissue, which will vary with different brain structures and different injuries.

When a person undergoes an MRI scan, he is placed in a large magnetic tube for 10 to 90 minutes. During that time his brain is pulsed with magnetism, and the resultant signals bounce back and are converted into visual images. No radiation is involved. Later, the images can be viewed in 3-D on a computer screen.

Because it provides such a high resolution of small changes, an MRI is more sensitive than the CAT scan in detecting small or early strokes, some tumors, and diseases like multiple sclerosis. Since the MRI is a magnetic field, these scans may not be possible in people with metal objects in their bodies such as cardiac pacemakers or clips around an aneurysm. Fortunately most hardware – plates, screws, and joint replacements – are unaffected by MRI.

In patients with dementia, an MRI may more accurately show the shrinking brain and empty spaces that used to be filled with brain tissue. An MRI can also show something called white matter disease, a condition where multiple small strokes have affected the connecting filaments coming off the brain cells. White matter disease in combination with the changes of Alzheimer's is a sure formula for dementia.

Mrs. Jones, in her seventies came to me because she couldn't balance, fell often, had stiff, poorly coordinated muscles and did not think clearly or remember well. She had become dependent on her husband to care for her. An MRI of her brain showed multiple small strokes, probably on the basis of a lifetime of hypertension that had only recently been brought under control. All we could do for this patient was get her a walker so she did not fall as often and control all her risks to prevent more strokes.

But the part of the story I wanted to tell you is that she has a lovely 50-year-old daughter, Linda. While Linda currently has no neurologic symptoms, she is concerned that she could suffer the same fate as her mother. I recommended that Linda see Dr. Felberg, our stroke specialist. He treated her with one baby aspirin a day, and one gram of fish oil per day. He also recommended a home blood pressure cuff (for the upper arm) so that if her blood pressure rose to 130/80 or more, Linda would alert us so that we could quickly bring it down with medicine. Dr. Felberg also emphasized to the daughter the extreme importance of daily aerobic exercise on a treadmill, stair stepper, or bicycle, or swimming for at least 30 minutes a day to dilate the tiny blood vessels to the brain.

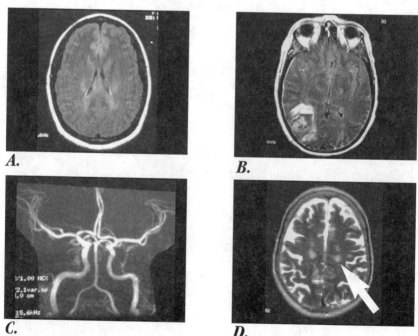

A. Normal MRI, B. MRI of a stroke victim, C. MRA of Normal Brain Blood supply,
D. White Matter Disease on an MRI.

I believe that by intervening early, we can prevent Linda from having small strokes. Linda is highly motivated to follow our recommendations after seeing what her mother went through.

Two areas of MRI research are functional and perfusion MRI. Functional MRI uses sophisticated software to show areas of the brain that are active while performing a mental task. Perfusion MRI can estimate blood flow to different brain regions.

MRA (magnetic resonance angiography) is designed to look at blood vessels in the brain. Using this technology doctors can see narrowed blood vessels that could potentially lead to stroke. An MRA is good for identifying aneurysms and may show an area where a short blockage is amenable to stenting to improve blood flow. If multiple blood vessels are narrowed, a patient may need to take Plavix, a strong blood thinner that helps prevent stroke.

Here is a good example of the use of an MRA study. Florence, a seventy-year-old woman had orthopedic surgery, and shortly thereafter had a stroke. Florence had no prior history of stroke or heart disease, was not a smoker and her blood pressure was well controlled with medicine. However, her MRA showed a short blockage in a single blood vessel, which supplies a major part of the right side of brain that controls the left side of the face, the left arm and leg. Once we had identified the problem, the interventional cardiologist was able to stent open the blockage and restore the blood flow. Although Florence had suffered damage to some of her brain cells during the stroke, she was able to be rehabilitated and go on living normally at home.

PET and SPECT Scans

The PET (positron emission tomography) scan, which measures the metabolic activity in the brain, remains largely a research tool for studying brain disease. To do this kind of scan, a technician injects a special radioactive-tagged sugar into the blood. The tagged sugar spreads throughout the brain in about a minute, and then the ring-shaped PET scanner records the radionuclide activity. When an area of the brain is active, it sucks up sugar at a rate related to the amount of activity. The scan shows the activity in different colors. Probable Alzheimer's can be seen early by PET scan as diminished brain activity.

SPECT (single photon emission computed tomography) also uses radionuclides (the radioactive sugar) to show blood flow to the brain. Once the radionuclide is injected into the blood, the scan can measure the greatest areas of blood flow by the highest number of counts.

PET and SPECT scans are not covered benefits of most insurance companies as tests for brain disease because they are considered expensive but may soon be covered. Medicare's worst nightmare is that all eligible people with dementia might want a PET or SPECT scan to find out more about a condition that so far is not that treatable. And what if serial expensive scans became the trend? At least for now, financial issues are one of several limitations that keep this technology from mainstream use. Their usefulness will have to be revisited when drugs that prevent the development of the plaques and tangles of Alzheimer's disease become available.

PET scans are more sensitive than SPECT scans for showing changes of Alzheimer's disease because metabolism slows down before blood flow decreases. Both PET and SPECT scans would show a probable diagnosis of Alzheimer's before brain changes showed on a CAT scan or an MRI. Brain shrinkage on CAT scan or MRI is seen later than slowed metabolism and decreased blood flow.

Let me tell you a remarkable story in which the combination of ultrasound, and PET scanning helped us identify a problem that would have occurred in ten or twenty years, enabling us to take steps to prevent dementia and stroke. The patient, Marie, is highly intelligent and generous. She said that if her story could help someone else, she wanted me to write about it in this book.

Ten years ago I was Marie's mother's doctor. Her mother smoked and drank heavily, and by her early sixties, had profound dementia. Most notably, she could no longer talk. Her basic brain function deteriorated steadily over the next two years. Finally she could not eat. The family decided not to force food with a feeding tube since they knew that would be against her wishes.

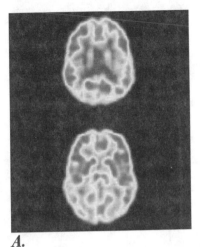 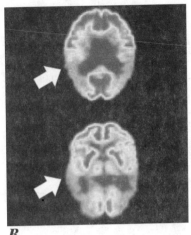

A. *B.*

A. Normal PET scan. B. PET scan in Alzheimer's. Arrows show absence of activity in memory area. (The top scans are at rest and the lower scans are with mental activity).

Several years after her mother died, Marie came to see at age 48. As I looked at her, I saw the same beauty and features that her mother had possessed. Marie had quit smoking two years earlier, although she still drank an average amount for some women who live in New Orleans. Her blood pressure was high at 150/70.

I had a bad feeling. Marie so resembled her mother that I began to worry that she would lose brain function in the next twenty years. I referred her to Dr. Felberg, an Ochsner Clinic expert in stroke. He often sees patients for me whom I identify as susceptible to stroke and dementia. Dr. Felberg did an ultrasound of all the blood vessels supplying her brain. Unfortunately, he found that at age 48, Marie already had a narrowed blood vessel to the most crucial part of the brain, that supplied by the left middle cerebral artery that controls speech; strength, movement and sensation on the right side of the body. My hunch was right…Marie's risk was great.

The next step was to request that Dr. Nachar, our nuclear medicine doctor do a SPECT scan to determine the blood flow to the brain. He found that the blood flow in the narrowed artery was still adequate, so Marie and her doctors could act now to prevent stroke. We advised her to take one coated baby aspirin a day, one gram of fish oil, 40 mg. of Pravachol, and we lowered her blood pressure with an ACE inhibitor medicine. In the rest of the book, I will review the rationale for each of these treatments. As Marie's doctor, I believe that by reversing the process of atherosclerotic narrowing of her blood vessels, we will prevent her from having a stroke.

A Functional Test for Dementia, the Mini-mental Status Exam

The Simple Version

Doctors and researchers commonly use the Mini-mental Status Exam to test for dementia. The test results are not always accurate because they vary according to age, education, and ethnicity.

The Details

The Mini-mental Status Exam takes a few minutes and can be performed during a routine office visit. This contrasts with detailed neuropsychological testing performed by a trained psychologist, which takes several hours to complete and expertise to interpret. Although widely used, the Mini-mental Status Exam often does not detect dementia because it asks questions to which almost anyone would know the answers. An intelligent and educated person can score perfectly even with dementia, while those with only an eighth grade education may score in the demented range, whether or not they have dementia. For this reason, test scores are adjusted for a person's educational level. Often, by the time an educated person does poorly on the Mini-mental Status Exam, their dementia is noticeable and they have already lost a lot of their brain function. Depressed people do not have the concentration to perform the test.

The modified Mini-mental Status Exam has 100 questions and is used more often in research. It is also considered to be only a screening device and not helpful in distinguishing the fine points of brain deficits.

Neuropsychological testing is a more detailed form of adult intellectual testing than the Mini-mental Status Exam. It checks for frontal brain function, those responses that make people civilized and give them judgment and socially acceptable behavior. Neuropsychological testing also checks for the ability to plan, to name things, and to store and remember new information. While full neuropsychological testing is better than the Mini-mental Status Exam for measuring dementia, it is still not infallible. I have witnessed highly intelligent people score well on this test while those who know them are certain that they are not mentally what they used to be.

Here is the Mini-mental Status Exam. An educated person must score over 28 points to be within normal range, and an uneducated person must score over 24.

Score	Interpretation
Less than 28, educated person	dementia
Less than 24, uneducated person	dementia
18-24	mild dementia
12-18	moderate dementia
Less than 12	more severe dementia

Mini-mental Status Exam:

Ask patient, "What is the year? Season, date, day, month?"
      0 out of 5 (0 points)
      1 out of 5 (1 point)
      2 out of 5 (2 points)
      3 out of 5 (3 points)
      4 out of 5 (4 points)
      5 out of 5 (5 points)

Ask patient, "Where are we? State, country, town, hospital, floor?"
      0 out of 5 (0 points)
      1 out of 5 (1 point)
      2 out of 5 (2 points)
      3 out of 5 (3 points)
      4 out of 5 (4 points)
      5 out of 5 (5 points)

Tell patient, "I'd like to test your memory;
say these words: boat, cucumber, wire"
      Says 0 out of 3 (0 points)
      Says 1 out of 3 (1 point)

Says 2 out of 3 (2 points)
Says 3 out of 3 (3 points)

Tell patient, "Begin with 100 and count backwards by 7"
Answers: (93, 86, 79, 72, 65)
Cannot do it at all (0 points)
Gets 1 right (1 point)
Gets 2 right (2 points)
Gets 3 right (3 points)
Gets 4 right (4 points)
Gets 5 right (5 points)

Tell patient, "Can you name the three objects I named before?"
Gets 0 out of 3 (0 points)
Gets 1 out of 3 (1 point)
Gets 2 out of 3 (2 points)
Gets all 3 (3 points)

Tell patient, "Name these items" and point to a pencil and a watch.
Gets neither one right (0 points)
Gets 1 of 2 right (1 point)
Gets them both right (2 points)

Tell patient, "Repeat the following: 'No ifs, ands or buts'."
Does not say it properly (0 points)
Says it properly (1 point)

Tell patient "Take a paper in your right hand,
fold it in half, and put it on the floor."
Does none of these 3 things (0 points)
Does 1 of these 3 things (1 point)
Does 2 of these 3 things (2 points)
Does 3 of these 3 things (3 points)

Tell the patient "Read and obey the following:
and write 'Close your eyes.'"

> Patient does not close eyes (0 points)
> Patient closes eyes (1 point)

Draw interlocking pentagons, and have patient copy it.

> Patient does not copy the design properly (0 points)
> Patient copies the design properly (1 point)

Why Is This Information About the Mini-mental Status Exam Important to You?

Within the next few years, you will be reading about studies of drugs purported to improve mental function or, in the case of the recent studies on estrogen and progesterone on brain function, decrease cognitive ability. If the only test that the researchers use is the Mini-mental Status Exam, then all you can really say is that these studies are inconclusive and that we need more information.

On the other hand, if a PET scan is used as an evaluation tool to test the effects of these drugs on people, then you can take the results of these studies seriously. The PET scan, which shows metabolism in different areas of the brain, at rest and while the brain is in action answering questions and remembering, is the gold standard test for Alzheimer's disease during life. PET scans can also pick up the earliest signs of dementia, before people even realize they have it. If a PET scan shows a drug increases brain metabolism, the drug may actually prevent Alzheimer's disease, provided the side-effects are tolerable.

Alzheimer's Disease

What Exactly Is Alzheimer's Disease?

The Simple Version

When we say Grandma had Alzheimer's disease, we need to be careful about what we are saying. A doctor cannot be absolutely sure that a patient had Alzheimer's without an autopsy after death that finds sticky microscopic plaques on the brain, useless tangles of nerve cells and a shrunken brain. Before death, all you can know is that someone has probable Alzheimer's. What most people call Alzheimer's disease is actually dementia, the loss of memory, social function, and cognitive ability. Dementia is brain failure. Alzheimer's is a specific type of brain failure.

The Details

Brain cells can either be killed, commit murder, or commit suicide. Causes of untimely death to brain cells include stroke where brain cells are suddenly starved for oxygen, head trauma, or alcohol or chemical abuse. When brain cells die from stroke or trauma, they release toxic signals to nearby brain cells and kill their neighbors. On the other hand, the suicide to which I refer is technically called apoptosis. All cells in the human body are programmed to die eventually, just as all humans seem programmed to die after their allotted years of life are up or all baby teeth are programmed to fall out in childhood. For reasons we do not understand, in some brain conditions, called neurodegenerative diseases, brain cells start to kill themselves early.

The signals that tell a cell to commit suicide are complex but scientists are unraveling them. Preventing the premature destruction of brain cells is the key to the cure for Alzheimer's, Parkinson's, Lou Gherig's disease, and other feared, irreversible neurologic diseases.

How Many People Have Dementia?

Dementia results from the progressive loss of nerve cells in the brain. People may live with dementia for two to 20 years. Two thirds of cases of dementia are attributed to Alzheimer's. Four million Americans have dementia now, and the number is expected to double or quadruple by 2050. About 1 percent of people between ages 65 and 69 are identified as having dementia and 40-50 percent will have it by age 95 as things are now.

Many more people probably have dementia than we know. Intelligent people can cover it up for many years by using wit. Adult children of an older parent living alone often say, "Mom (or Dad) is just fine." But upon what are they basing this assessment of their parent's mental acuity? Their interactions are usually repetitions of familiar behaviors. The extent of their communication may only be a quick telephone conversation with that older parent, once every few weeks. Rarely do they actually sit down with their parent to listen or to have anything like a detailed discussion. Mildly demented people often do remarkably well when their interactions are familiar and scripted.

Often, dementia is only discovered when something stressful or out of the ordinary happens – a hospitalization or a change in a prescription medicine, for instance. Suddenly the older person seems clearly confused and out of his or her element. In these situations, it is common for the children to assert once again, "But Mom was just fine until this happened." The truth of the matter is, Mom was slowly developing dementia for years, and she has been living on the edge, compensating for her loss of memory and mental function in the restricted environment of her familiar surroundings.

We see this all too often when an older woman falls and breaks her hip. While in the hospital, she gets disoriented. She has no idea what's happened to her; no idea where she is or why she's there. Before the hospitalization, her social functioning may have seemed fine to those around her, but she hadn't been challenged by complex concepts or conversations for a number of years. She lived well within the familiar, but had slowly lost her ability to cope with the unfamiliar – an early sign of dementia. Her confusion in the hospital shows that she was already developing dementia which was compensated before the accident.

I see this commonly when an elderly patient comes to the clinic for a pre-operative medical check-up prior to some major surgery – knee replacement, let's say. The patient is accompanied to the clinic by her daughter. After introducing myself and establishing some rapport with the patient and daughter, I begin asking questions about Mom's medical history. The patient is pleasant, but slow to answer. The daughter almost immediately chimes in, supplying the answers for her mother. After a few more questions, a pattern develops in which it's clear to me that if Mom had to answer these questions herself, she simply couldn't. I then politely ask the daughter to let her mother answer the next few questions, so that I can also get an idea of how her memory is working. This is particularly critical to me, since the risk of post-operative confusion is high after the stress of knee replacement – especially in a compensated, but already demented patient. And a patient who is confused after an elective operation that requires extensive therapy and rehabilitation is unlikely to get a good result. I may proceed from there to some simple questions such as asking her to remember three objects and then coming back a few minutes later in the interview to ask what those were. It isn't at all difficult to unmask dementia in these patients, but it can be surprising and embarrassing to both the patient and the family, so it has to be done carefully and with the utmost respect.

As a rule, doctors are not aggressive about diagnosing cases of dementia because there is so little that can be done about it once the syndrome is established. No more than 1.5 percent of cases of dementia of any kind are fully reversible.

Three Phases of Intellectual Decline
Decline in thinking ability with age has been categorized into:

- Age-associated memory impairment (AAMI), usually not a precursor to dementia
- Mild cognitive impairment (MCI), probably a precursor to dementia
- Dementia or probable Alzheimer's

Patients with AAMI may complain of memory loss but do well on neuropsychological (adult IQ) tests. Most of these people do not progress to dementia, although some do. The slowed speed of brain processing is expected with age.

Mildly cognitively impaired individuals (MCI) also complain of memory loss, but they have abnormal neuropsychological tests. Up to half will have dementia within three years and this condition is probably in the middle of the spectrum between normal and dementia. Poor sleep, depression, agitation, and apathy commonly accompany MCI. Treatment of these emotional problems may help patients function better, although there is no proof yet that it delays the onset of frank dementia.

Alzheimer's Disease

(Probable) Alzheimer's is usually a slow process in which it takes years to get to the earliest noticeable stages of the disease. At first, victims become forgetful and have difficulty with their job and household tasks. The first function they lose is the ability to form new memories. The victim cannot remember what was said to him or her just a moment ago. A few years later they forget names for simple things like silverware, lose the ability to use numbers, become spatially disoriented, lose interest in things they may have always enjoyed, and stop taking initiative. Their judgment wanes. So often I have seen these patients wearing dirty clothes and not realizing it.

As the disease progresses, patients fail to recognize family members, wander about and get lost, are confused and anxious, and cannot brush their teeth or dress themselves. When dementia is severe and the whole brain is involved, patients cannot process new information, use words, eat, swallow, control bladder and bowel function, or get out of bed.

In 1906 Dr. Alois Alzheimer, a German neuropathologist, first described this brain disease following the autopsy of a 55-year-old demented woman. This disease can appear as early as midlife in some unfortunate families that have a clear-cut genetic predisposition. However, almost everyone will have a few changes of Alzheimer's in their brain by the time they are eighty, but not all will become demented.

The research into the biochemistry and genetics of these brain changes is aggressive because the prevention of this disease could be worth billions of dollars to the pharmaceutical companies. The medicines presently available do only a little to ameliorate the symptoms of established dementia, but prevention is where the heavy-duty research is directed.

Researchers presently believe that amyloid plaques damage brain cells. The amyloid-beta 42 protein that comprises these plaques begins as a by-product of a normal protein, the amyloid-precursor protein (APP) that is attached to the brain cell's membrane. There are several chemical pathways in the formation of damaging amyloid-beta 42 protein, and each step could be blocked by a preventive drug if researchers could develop one and find a way to transmit it to the brain. The enzymes beta and gamma secretase generate this damaging amyloid residue from the APP, and their inhibition may prevent Alzheimer's.

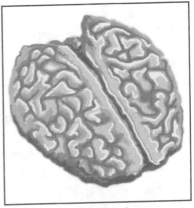

Normal, healthy brain

A vaccine against amyloid plaque is another approach. Such a vaccine was successful in dissolving amyloid plaque in laboratory animals, but the drug was toxic to normal tissues in humans. This will be the challenge for all future treatments: to prevent amyloid plaque without collateral damage. We also want to dissolve existing plaques, or to make them less sticky to brain cells. It is likely that in years to come, a PET scan, SPECT scan, or

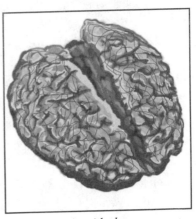

Brain with plaques and tangles of Alzheimer's

a functional and perfusion MRI will screen for toxic brain amyloid plaques at midlife. If it appears that Alzheimer's is in a person's future, he or she will gladly take preventive medicine.

What about those suicidal brain cells? Proteins called caspases are being studied for their role in causing brain cells to commit suicide. If a way to block the negative effects of caspases can be found, then brain cells can be prevented from killing themselves in a number of neurologic diseases.

The last problem to be solved are the tangles that are seen at autopsy in Alzheimer's disease. Each brain cell is nourished by a long, railroad-like strand that emanates from it. These strands, which contain a protein called TAU, twist and become useless, causing the tangles that are a hallmark of Alzheimer's. Can TAU, the molecule that supports the nerve cell's nourishing projections, be protected so that the strands do not become useless tangles?

Snowdon states in his book, *Aging With Grace,* that he believes these TAU tangles are the cause of brain damage in Alzheimer's. The autopsies conducted in the Nun Study showed that the distribution and density of the TAU tangles in the sisters who died closely matched the severity of their dementia. But it is the additive effect of multiple small brain injuries superimposed on varying degrees of Alzheimer's changes in the aging brain that causes dementia, that final common pathway of brain failure.

Location of Alzheimer's in the Brain

Alzheimer's tangles first begin in a region near the base of the skull, the entorhinal cortex that is necessary for memory. Next they appear in the hippocampus, another area where we learn and remember new things. This distribution of disease probably accounts for the early impairment of short term memory. The condition of the hippocampus is critical in Alzheimer's. One of the characteristics of Alzheimer's on a PET scan is decreased metabolism in both the right and left hippocampus. Later on in the disease, one sees shrunken lobes of the hippocampus.

At the end, the plaques and tangles reach the neocortex, the highly developed gray matter unique to humans. We take the functions of the neocortex for granted – telling time, being oriented in space, making decisions, interpreting sights and sounds. When those brain cells are destroyed, the simplest parts of living are also gone.

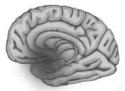 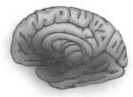 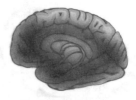

1. Early Stage   2. Middle Stage   3. Late Stage

1. Alzheimer's tangles first begin in the entorhinal cortex. 2. Next they appear in the hippocampus. 3. Finally, the plaques and tangles reach the neocortex.

Genetic Susceptibility to Alzheimer's Disease

The Simple Version

Genetics vs. environment and nature vs. nurture…when it comes to dementia, those are still huge unanswered questions.

The Details

APOE-4 is the gene associated with old age Alzheimer's. As we discussed in the Nun Study, you can inherit one or two copies of this gene. If you have one APOE-4 gene, whether or not you get dementia in your lifetime probably depends on a number of factors under your control such as stroke, head trauma, toxins, and how you conduct your life. Having one APOE-4 gene is not a diagnostic test for Alzheimer's disease, just for the predisposition later in life. However, the one in fifty people who have two APOE-4 genes are more likely to get dementia in their lifetime, no matter what they do.

Fourteen percent of white Americans have at least one copy of the APOE-4 gene. Thirty percent of patients who develop classic symptoms of Alzheimer's disease (later documented by autopsy) do not carry the APOE-4 gene. A person with one copy of APOE-4 may get dementia 5 to 10 years earlier than someone without a copy, and a person with two copies of APOE-4 may get manifestations of the disease 10 to 20 years earlier than his peers. I have seen unfortunate patients with dementia in their 50's who have two APOE-4 genes.

On the other hand, another gene, the APOE-2 gene, may protect a person from Alzheimer's. Clearly there is more to this story.

I did not want to use examples of dementia because the purpose of this book is teach brain protection, not to tell one sad story after another. But I must also point out that some cases of dementia are clearly genetic and therefore not under a person's control. I had a 59-year-old patient, Phil, a few weeks ago who previously functioned at a high level with complex concepts. His ability to think, remember, and talk had gradually diminished over three years. His neurologist's findings were most consistent with pure Alzheimer's disease, not stroke or any other dementing condition. The neurologist checked Phil's APOE-4 genetic status because it was crucial to get the diagnosis right. Unfortunately, Phil had two APOE-4 genes, and did indeed have early onset Alzheimer's. As of now, doctors cannot offer him a cure and the goal is to help him function as well as he can. He can no longer work and is on disability.

There are some other rare genes that cause Alzheimer's disease listed below. If people have these genes, or two copies of APOE-4, they cannot prevent Alzheimer's disease. However, less than 10 percent of people carrying these genes develop early-onset Alzheimer's before the age of 65. Conversely, about 7 percent of these early-onset cases are inherited.

At least 72 genetic variants have been identified that cause Alzheimer's sticky amyloid plaques. A mutant gene on chromosome #21 causes less than 1 percent of Alzheimer's cases, with symptoms beginning between the ages of 45 and 65. Presenilin-1 on chromosome #14 causes 4 percent of cases, with symptoms beginning between the ages of 28 and 50, and presenilin-2 on chromosome #1 probably causes 1 percent of the cases that develop between the ages of 40 and 50. Just hope that you and your family are not among these unfortunate genetic carriers.

Depression and Dementia

The Simple Version

Depression and dementia go hand in hand. It can be hard to tell the chicken from the egg.

The Details

Depression is more common in older people with dementia than in normal folks. Anyone who has experienced even mild depression knows that the feeling is not just a loss of morale but, at times, a loss of mind. The incidence of depression in those with probable Alzheimer's is between 15 and 40 percent.

On one hand, depression causes loss of concentration. Some older adults, when treated for depression, can recover a modicum of their former selves. On the other hand, if a person has dementia, there may be no way to overcome his or her depression and return to normal. The reason for this is that the parts of the brain that allow us emotional expression may become blunted with the dementing disease. We all know people whose entire personality changed when they were stricken, reasonable people who became irrational and paranoid, socially well-behaved persons who turned into screamers and cursors, and formerly animated, creative people who became speechless.

So, dementia causes emotional changes by its very nature. We glibly assume that the demented people don't recall enough of their former selves to be depressed by their condition, but those with early dementia do seem to know that things aren't right. They know that something major, life-altering, and beyond their control is happening to them, and that can be depressing. We also see irritability, apathy, and agitation as common emotional symptoms of dementia.

Then there is the question that was so significantly raised by The Nun Study. When does Alzheimer's – and its accompanying depression – really begin (as opposed to when do people and their loved ones know they have it)? If this disease starts in the early twenties, is someone with chronic depression in reality manifesting a brain inefficiency that worsens over a lifetime? Efficient brain and emotional centers allow people to cope, forgive, distinguish between what they can and cannot do anything about, attract and maintain love relationships and friendships, and raise happy children. If a person's brain isn't functioning properly, he or she may be chronically angry, upset, carry grudges, project faults onto others, and have more negative than positive emotions.

The standard of care in psychiatry and medicine is to treat depressed people with medicine so that their condition does not worsen. Many patients have experienced an amazing turn around with the anti-depressants known as selective serotonin reuptake inhibitors (SSRIs) that have become available over the last twenty years. Of course, there are questions about use of these medicines. How long should people take anti-depressants, for a short time or a long time? If we think about the long term, do anti-depressants have a good effect on mental function later in life for those with inefficient brains, or could they in some way be detrimental by altering brain chemistry in some people? When we correct depression, do we prevent dementia in those with genetic susceptibility, such as one copy of the APOE-4 gene? No one knows.

We really can't analyze brain chemistry in living humans. By the time they are deceased, the chemistry of the living brain is no longer functioning or analyzable. By then all an autopsy can show is the damage the brain has sustained physically. So we have a lot of unknowns about anti-depressants even though they are widely used and people seem to do much better with the medicine.

Other Conditions That Cause Dementia
I have a theory that President Ronald Reagan's primary problem was not Alzheimer's disease. Rather, he suddenly lost half his blood during the 1981 assassination attempt, and I suspect he did not get enough oxygen to his brain. I believe it was this insult (technically called anoxic encephalopathy) that caused this intelligent man to get dementia later on.

There are other physical problems that mimic the effects of Alzheimer's. Small strokes that go unnoticed can result in decreased mentation. Other brain diseases like Crueztfeldt-Jakob, which is similar to mad cow disease; Lewy body dementia, which causes visual hallucinations and dementia; Pick's disease, which affects different parts of the brain than Alzheimer's, and Parkinson's disease are all recognized as destroyers of brain function by pathologists who examine the brain. Head trauma can cause dementia. For example, boxers' brains may shrink from repeated blows to the head. The brain damage from alcoholism significantly affects memory and intellect. At autopsy, all of these different brain diseases and injuries show the distinctive signs of the build-up of amyloid plaques.

Diseases in other parts of the body can undermine clear mental functioning. Heart failure, emphysema and its accompanying oxygen deprivation, an underactive thyroid, a low sodium level in the blood, and severe sleep apnea are a few of these.

A vitamin B12 deficiency may cause dementia and other symptoms such as loss of balance, although replacing it does not seem to restore mental function in older people. The vitamin B12 level is measured in the blood, not directly in the neurologic tissue. However if it is borderline low in the blood test, we must assume it is lower than normal in the neurologic tissue. Usually, a B12 deficiency occurs when a person has difficulty absorbing vitamin B12 from food. The absorption of B12 from food can be decreased in people taking drugs such as Prilosec, Nexium and similar medicine for heartburn which reduces stomach acid although most people taking these medications still get enough B12. Pernicious anemia means that the protein that allows B12 to get into the blood is no longer made in the stomach. If a person has a low B12 level, this vitamin is replaced by monthly injections or B12 tablets under the tongue.

In older adults who are often taking multiple medicines, doctors must always be aware of possible drug interactions and side-effects. Some medicines that wouldn't faze a younger person may make an older person confused. I include in this list tranquilizers, sleeping pills (including those sold over-the-counter), anti-depressants, some blood pressure medicines, cold remedies, and pain medicines.

When a patient sees the doctor for cognitive impairment, the doctor usually does a history, physical exam, and blood tests for anemia, blood chemistries, liver, kidney and thyroid function. The patient may have a brain CAT scan, neuropsychological testing, and a neurology consultation. This book is aimed at preserving the brain cells, not what to do once they are damaged. That is a whole other story.

Causes of Dementia Other Than Alzheimer's

- Small unrecognized strokes (also called white matter disease)
- Parkinson's disease
- Drug or alcohol abuse
- Sudden loss of oxygen to the brain (anoxic encephalopathy due to the heart stopping or loss of blood)
- Head trauma
- Other rare brain diseases: Crueztfeldt-Jakob (similar to mad cow disease), Lewy body dementia, Pick's disease, AIDS encephalopathy
- Other diseases such as heart failure, low blood sodium, under-active thyroid and low vitamin B12 levels
- Side-effects of medicine

What Can You Do To Prevent Dementia?

The Simple Version

Here is the down-and-dirty prescription if you want to preserve brain function as you age. You are less likely to get dementia if you exercise aerobically every day, don't smoke, and take blood pressure medicine if necessary to keep your blood pressure under 130/80. Try to avoid injury to your brain by always wearing your seatbelt when you drive, having someone stand there and watch you if you have to get on a ladder, wearing a helmet when bicycling or riding a motorcycle; and avoiding activities that are dangerous, such as contact sports. Don't put your brain at risk.

The Details

Think of dementia as a bell shaped curve. No one at age 100 is going to be as quick as he or she was at age 25. However you probably can move back the time you might get dementia by ten years if you learn how to protect and maintain your brain function. If that means you will be 120-years-old when you are susceptible to dementia, that is not a threat. Even if you are one of those people who will get dementia during your lifetime, your symptoms do not have to be annihilating and devastating if you keep your brain and body as healthy as possible. Fortunately, dementia is one of those serious, common diseases where there are many things you can do to help yourself. The key phrase here is "help yourself." Doctors can't give you a pill to preserve your brain function; you must choose a lifestyle that preserves your brain.

Exercise prevents dementia. Regular aerobic exercise means sustained walking at 3 to 4 miles an hour, running, cycling, swimming or other activities that raise your pulse rate over 110 and make you hot and sweaty. Researchers believe that physical exercise prevents cognitive decline by increasing blood flow to the brain. Exercise may also stimulate the growth of brain cells. Because exercise is healthy for almost every part of the body, you should take this prescription seriously.

One of the most important things you can do to prevent dementia is to stop smoking. Smoking is highly toxic to the brain cells and the blood vessels that supply them.

Keeping Your Blood Pressure Less Than 130/80 May Prevent Dementia.

High blood pressure is definitely associated with dementia, whether through direct damage to brain cells or because it narrows and closes the fine blood vessels that supply oxygen and nutrients to these cells. Blood pressure can be lowered with weight loss, exercise, and sometimes a low salt diet. Often, it takes medicine to lower blood pressure.

Two Types of Medicine That May Prevent Dementia

Cholesterol-lowering and anti-inflammatory medicines may prevent dementia. Cholesterol-lowering medicine reduces the risk of stroke and probably interferes with the formation of those sticky amyloid plaques. Anti-inflammatory medicine such as ibuprofen turns off the immune cells in the body. Immune cells may attack not only unwanted bacteria that try to invade the body, but they may also attack blood vessels with atherosclerosis and brain cells with amyloid plaque.

A few small recent studies showed that two cholesterol-lowering drugs, in the group of medicine called the statins, Pravachol (pravastatin) and Zocor (simstatin), may prevent dementia. The entire class of statin drugs may have the same effect because the APOE-4 gene seen in Alzheimer's victims is related to cholesterol. Statins probably reduce the number and size of sticky amyloid plaques on the brain. In one study, people taking statins had a 39 percent decrease in the risk of Alzheimer's. If further studies bear out these earlier findings, this is significant information. We may all want to take a statin not only to prevent a heart attack and stroke, but also to prevent dementia.

Statins work by blocking the liver enzyme that manufactures cholesterol. Statins also decrease inflammation in cells lining blood vessels and help the liver remove LDL cholesterol (the bad kind) more efficiently from the bloodstream.

In addition to the plaques stuck to the brain and the useless tangles of former nerve connections, the brains at autopsy of Alzheimer's victims also have inflammatory cells, those same cells that make arthritic joints swell or cause fever during a bout of tonsillitis. This inflammation may damage even more brain cells. Anti-inflammatory drugs block inflammation and therefore they may also help prevent dementia. There are some studies purporting to show an association between taking these drugs and having less dementia, but this association is not yet scientifically verified. Given how slowly dementia develops and how late in life people discover that they have it, a study comparing those who use anti-inflammatory medicine and those who do not would have to go on for many years. For now, I consider it possible that taking an Advil a few times a week will help prevent brain cell damage from Alzheimer's disease.

How Stroke and
Alzheimer's Disease
Cause Dementia Together

The Simple Version

What I say in this short chapter is the single most important concept in this book. People tend to be fatalistic about whether they will get dementia. Yet they do not realize how important the connection is between stroke and dementia – and what they can do to avoid stroke.

Whereas the changes of Alzheimer's are not preventable, stroke is largely preventable. The risks for stroke, abnormal cholesterol, hypertension and smoking are within your control. If you have both stroke and Alzheimer's, you are much more likely to be demented. If you can avoid stroke, even if you have the gene for late life Alzheimer's, you may be able to delay the onset of dementia until something else takes you from this world.

The Details

They used to call it hardening of the arteries. During the first seventy years of the twentieth century, doctors believed that dementia was caused by lack of blood supply to the brain just like heart attacks were caused by poor circulation.

In the 1970's, the medical establishment changed its collective mind and decided there were basically two common kinds of dementia, Alzheimer's, which was gradual and progressive, and strokes or cerebrovascular disease, which caused sudden, episodic damage. When a patient had a stroke, he took a step down.

But real patients didn't easily fall into categories of gradual versus stepwise mental deterioration. And with more recent studies, including PET scans and autopsy findings correlated with neuropsychological testing, we now believe that the changes of Alzheimer's in the brain don't always cause dementia unless accompanied by strokes, especially small strokes aimed at the white matter (nerve connections) of the brain. Similarly, even though stroke causes specific deficits, stroke doesn't cause dementia unless changes of Alzheimer's are also present. Furthermore, there is a striking overlap in the conditions that cause both stroke and dementia. Hypertension, high cholesterol, smoking, diabetes, and high homocysteine are serious risks for both conditions.

If an MRI of the brain is done in older people and they are found to have more than one silent small stroke, their chance of being demented is greatly increased.

Here are some theories on why stroke and Alzheimer's changes work together to cause dementia. Decreased blood flow caused by strokes enhances damage to brain cells from Alzheimer's disease by depriving the cells of oxygen and nutrients. Conversely, perhaps Alzheimer's disease, the presence of plaques and tangles, makes nerve cells more vulnerable to damage from a temporary drop in blood flow. A brain with Alzheimer's disease may be able to compensate by using other circuits unless these other pathways have been cut off by stroke.

The Nun Study clearly showed that stroke and Alzheimer's are most commonly found together at the brain autopsy of patients with dementia. The extent of dementia was carefully documented throughout the later lives of these aging sisters. Then autopsies of the brain were done. If the brain had enough plaques and tangles to diagnose Alzheimer's, then the addition of small strokes and atherosclerosis of blood vessels in the brain almost certainly caused dementia while the nun was alive.

What is Stroke?

The Simple Version

Stroke is brain cell death due to a sudden loss of blood flow to part of the brain. Untreated hypertension, and smoking are two of the main causes of stroke.

The Details

Just as high blood pressure and smoking damage the heart, they damage the brain. Though the heart is accessible to vascular bypass and even transplant – the same cannot be said of the brain. Infarcted heart muscle (i.e., that damaged by poor blood flow) may self-repair or continue to function, but if you deprive brain cells of their oxygen, they are gone forever.

Stroke is the third most common cause of death in this country after heart attack and cancer. Each year more than 600,000 Americans suffer a stroke. Although about 160,000 persons die of stroke annually, death is not the worst consequence of this disease. Rather, the long-term disability, helplessness, and dependence on others for basic needs are the most feared outcomes.

Stroke Can Happen in Several Different Ways:

- Obstruction of large and/or small blood vessels (ischemic stroke)
- Hemorrhage from rupture of a brain blood vessel and bleeding into the tissue outside it
- Embolus, a blood clot that forms elsewhere, travels through blood vessels to those that supply the brain, and blocks the blood flow to the brain

What Is a Mini-stroke?

I try to avoid the term mini-stroke because patients use it to mean two different things. Some people think it means a transient ischemic attack or a TIA, a temporary blocked blood flow to a part of the brain with temporary neurologic deficiency. A TIA clears when the blood flow is spontaneously restored, but it can be a warning that a larger permanent stroke is on the way. However, it is also true that MRI examinations of patients who were thought to have had a TIA show about that about half of these individuals have already had a completed stroke – there was nothing temporary about it.

The term mini-stroke is also used by patients to describe multiple small strokes of which they are unaware. In this case, the term "mini" is far from accurate. This is indeed a scary phenomenon because it leads to serious brain damage over time.

For the sake of accuracy, we will call multiple small strokes small vessel disease (the underlying cause of small strokes) and/or white matter disease (what radiologists call this when they see it on an MRI).

Warning Signs of Stroke Include:
- Loss of vision in one eye
- Loss of speech
- Numbness on one side of the body or in one limb
- Weakness on one side of the body
- Double vision

The Role of Cholesterol in Stroke
When cholesterol, a waxy solid substance is functioning in a healthy way, it works as a building block for the membranes of cells and the sex hormones. Lipoproteins transport cholesterol in the blood. Low-density lipoprotein (LDL, also known as the bad kind of cholesterol) moves cholesterol from the liver to atherosclerotic deposits in blood vessels. High-density lipoprotein (HDL, the good kind of cholesterol) moves cholesterol out of blood vessels back to the liver to be discarded.

Ischemic Stroke
Ischemia means loss of blood supply. Atherosclerosis may progressively narrow blood vessels all over the body causing the build-up of cholesterol-laden plaque and the thickening of the tiny muscle cells in blood vessels when they are stressed by high blood pressure. If the blood vessels leading directly to the heart close, a person will experience a heart attack. If the blood vessels to the penis narrow, a man will experience impotence. If the inflow to the legs is blocked, that person will experience pain, perhaps leg ulcers, or, in the worst case scenario, an amputation. If the blood vessels to the brain narrow or close, it may cause stroke.

A blood vessel may also close suddenly when an atherosclerotic plaque becomes unstable. Most people think that the cholesterol plaque that builds up in the blood vessels is like the bark of a tree that adds a layer every year, narrowing the vessel progressively. Instead, it is a dynamic chemical milieu that changes over time. If the plaque ruptures, platelets rush to the site and clump up to stop bleeding, just as they would at the site of any small cut on the body. Because a blood vessel is such a small space, the clump of platelets blocks off the flow of blood. This is called a thrombus. So, it is often the thrombus that causes the stroke.

Ischemic Stroke in the Blood Vessels Leading to the Brain

Simplistically speaking, the right side of the brain controls feeling and strength on the left side of the body, and the left side of the brain controls the usually dominant right side of the body, including the speech center. Different brain tasks are located throughout the brain, which is why certain strokes, depending on their location and size, can cause unusual selected disabilities. Antoine's syndrome, for example, is a stroke near the back of the brain that renders a patient blind without knowing he is blind.

Four large blood vessels carry all the blood to the brain, the two carotid arteries in the front of the neck, and the two vertebral arteries that run through pathways inside the bone of the cervical spine at the back of the neck. Depending on which large vessel closes, the result is most often a large stroke with sudden paralysis and numbness on one side of the body, or loss of speech, eyesight, or balance. In extreme cases, a person will lose of awareness of one half of the body.

These four large vessels are all connected by the Circle of Willis, a circular flow of blood at the base (lowest part) of the brain. This allows blood flow from one vessel to augment that in another. If there is atherosclerosis in the Circle of Willis blocking this cross flow, Dr. Snowdon notes the increased risk of dementia in the nuns he studied.

If the blood flow is slowed in the large vessels due to partial blockage, blood may flow slowly, then stagnate and clot in the fine blood vessels branching off the larger ones, resulting in white matter or small-vessel disease. These debilitating strokes affect the white matter, those long communication strands off the nerve cells. Gradually, a person with this kind of problem will lose neurologic functions such as fine coordination, ease of gait, regulation of muscle tension, and mental acuity.

Hemorrhagic and Embolic Stroke

Less commonly, a stroke results from a hemorrhage when a blood vessel ruptures in the brain and spills blood onto adjacent brain cells, disrupting their blood supply and function. This kind of stroke can happen in several ways. An aneurysm, for example, is the result of a blood vessel with a thin wall that balloons and suddenly bursts, causing a subarachnoid hemorrhage at any age in adults. In older adults, a hemorrhagic stroke can occur when a small blood vessel that has been under too much pressure, heart beat by heart beat, bursts suddenly. Tiny weak spots in the brain's delicate blood vessels caused by high blood pressure can also result in microscopic hemorrhages and swelling of the brain.

Atrial fibrillation, an abnormal heart rhythm in a weak heart, causes blood stasis and clots in the heart chambers. The clots, called emboli, may move to the brain.

Types of Strokes
- Large vessel atherosclerosis
- Small vessel atherosclerosis (white matter disease)
- Large hemorrhage
- Multiple small hemorrhages from uncontrolled hypertension
- Embolus

Will You Always Know that You Have Had a Stroke?

No, not always. If a stroke victim is asleep, he or she may not notice a subtle difference in brain function. If no one usually expects much from them, including themselves, they may not be aware of losing function. Also, collateral circulation from other blood vessels may step in and supply brain cells if their primary source of blood and oxygen collapses.

So, many strokes are unrecognized. The reason this matters is that one stroke is a significant risk factor for another. And unrecognized strokes correlate strongly with cognitive decline.

Other Factors Causing Stroke: Homocysteine and C-reactive Protein

In recent years, two new factors have emerged that can put healthy blood vessels at risk. The first is homocysteine an amino acid, a building block of protein that all animals produce naturally. A high homocysteine level predisposes a person to stroke because it is toxic to the cells lining blood vessels – and probably also toxic to brain cells.

C-reactive protein is another measure of propensity to atherosclerosis. If you have an elevated, highly sensitive C-reactive protein, which is a marker of inflammation, what does that mean for you? Ideally, the immune system identifies and destroys foreign bacteria or viruses in the body, but sometimes a person's own cells may be misidentified as "foreign" and be battered by the "friendly fire" of the body's own immune cells, a condition known as inflammation. This is the same confusion between friend and foe that accounts for diseases like rheumatoid arthritis and lupus. We also think that chronic bacterial infections may contribute to atherosclerosis by directly infecting blood vessels or through inflammation.

Stroke under Age 60

Stroke is usually the result of lifestyle factors and age. So, if a patient suffers a stroke under the age of 60, he or she will often have an unusual underlying cause. For example, if the patient's blood clots too easily, as happens in some inherited blood disorders, his or her brain cells will be at risk. Vasculitis, a disease that directly inflames the blood vessels, may also cause stroke in these individuals.

An ophthalmologist consulted me about a thirty-seven-year-old, Matt, an otherwise healthy, non-smoking man in whom he had diagnosed a stroke causing sudden loss of vision in one eye. I checked Matt for unusual causes of stroke. Sure enough, he had both a high level of homocysteine, and another abnormal blood clotting factor called an antiphospholipid antibody (also known as lupus anti-coagulant).

One of the advantages to working at a medical center like Ochsner Clinic Foundation with so many specialists is that we can each look at a complex problem from the vantage point of different specialty training. I referred Matt to one of our hematologists who specializes in blood clotting disorders. The hematologist treated his high homocysteine with folic acid and prescribed life-long Coumadin (warfarin) to thin his blood and prevent a stroke in the other eye or in other areas of Matt's brain.

Lifestyle Changes Can Prevent Stroke
Since stroke is at least in part preventable, minimizing your risk of stroke is one of the most important things you can do to prevent dementia. I urge you to stop smoking; take your hypertension seriously and get it treated; exercise; and, if you have a family history of stroke, get checked for inherited, treatable causes like a clotting disorder or high homocysteine.

Before we move on to hypertension let's review some of the health risks and substances that can predispose you to stroke.

Risks That Predispose You to Stroke:
- Hypertension (blood pressure higher than 130/80)
- Deconditioning, lack of physical fitness
- High cholesterol and low HDL cholesterol
- Diabetes
- High homocysteine
- Elevated highly sensitive C-reactive protein
- Blood clotting disorders
- Heart failure
- Atrial fibrillation
- Family history of stroke
- Having already had a first stroke
- Coronary artery disease, blood vessel disease of the legs, and atherosclerosis

Substances that Can Cause Stroke:
- Cigarettes

- Alcohol in excess
- Cocaine
- Amphetamines
- Ephedrine
- Ma huang

Websites that give helpful information about strokes and stroke prevention are www.strokeassociation.org and http://209.107.44.93/NationalStroke/HavingAStroke

Hypertension

The Simple Version

First, let's get our terms right. Hypertension and high blood pressure are the same thing and doctors and patients use the terms interchangeably. Let me tell you right up front why hypertension matters. If your blood pressure is greater than 130/80 consistently, it damages brain cells and their blood supply, and makes you dull-witted in old age. If your mental abilities matter to you, then your blood pressure should matter to you.

The Details

Several large studies, in which people were observed over many years show that long-term untreated hypertension is strongly related to dementia. The famous Framingham, Massachusetts study is one of the best known. The relationship is even stronger in diabetics who also have hypertension. Research is in progress to show whether controlling blood pressure in older adults can improve mental function. But for the purpose of this book, the point is to normalize your blood pressure now while your brain is healthy.

There's a lot of folklore about hypertension and its treatment. Many patients still believe that it is related to stress (high tension) and that the medicines that treat it cause impotence, fatigue and other side-effects. Hypertension does not mean high emotional tension. It is not a mental state, nor is it mainly due to stress. It is a physical condition. If your parents had it you are more likely to have it. It is multifactorial, having to do with the "thermostat" in the brainstem that sets the blood pressure; the resistance in the blood vessels, which become stiffer with age; and certain hormones (the critically important angiotensin and renin) secreted by the kidneys, heart and blood vessels.

A normal blood pressure is less than 120/80 and prehypertension is a blood pressure of 120-139/80-89, measured in millimeters of mercury (mmHg). Blood pressure varies throughout the day. More physical activity temporarily raises blood pressure. The top number is the systolic pressure generated as the heart beats and the bottom number is the diastolic pressure when the heart relaxes after a heart beat. Both are important and need to be normalized.

High blood pressure often starts between age 30 and 50. An increasing number of people develop it as they age so that by age 60 at least one third of people have high blood pressure. If your blood pressure is normal now, check it every year just in case it takes a turn for the worse. If you have a family history of hypertension, stroke, or heart attack, you must be particularly vigilant. Keep a record of when your blood pressure was last checked, and when it should be checked again (within one year if it is normal, more frequently if it is high or you take anti-hypertensive medicine). Do not depend upon your doctor to call you in for a blood pressure check. You may change health insurance plans, you may move, or your doctor could die, lose his memory, or have a stroke himself.

Blood Pressure Categories

Ideal:	less than 120/80
High normal (prehypertension):	130-139/80-89
High:	greater than 140/90
Stage 1 hypertension:	140-159/90-99
Stage 2 hypertension:	160-179/100-109
Stage 3 hypertension:	Greater than 185/110

So, high blood pressure itself is not so much the problem as its effect on organs such as the brain, heart and kidneys. Patients with untreated hypertension often experience subtle symptoms of non-well-being such as fatigue, headache, shortness of breath and sexual dysfunction. They may not know that these symptoms are due to their high blood pressure. If an echocardiogram (ultrasound of the heart) shows a thickened heart muscle, called left ventricular hypertrophy, it means the person with hypertension is more likely to have a stroke or heart attack. Similarly, if the urine contains protein, it means that the kidneys are being damaged by hypertension. If a CAT scan or MRI of the brain shows small strokes, the brain damage has already begun.

Causes of Hypertension
- Obesity
- Genetics
- Too much salt in the diet (in some but not in all hypertensive patients)
- Increased resistance in blood vessels as one ages

- A higher set level of blood pressure determined by the deep structures of the brain
- Less commonly, a blocked renal artery or an adrenalin tumor, a tumor in the adrenal gland, that is constantly causing a "flight or fight" reaction

Medicine that Raises Blood Pressure

Over-the-counter decongestants such as Sudafed may raise blood pressure as do prescription decongestants that are often found in combination with an anti-allergy antihistamine such as Claritin-D, Allegra-D, and Zyrtec-D. The reason for this is that decongestants may act like an adrenalin surge.

Anti-inflammatory medicine for arthritis such as Motrin or Alleve and prescription arthritis medicine may also elevate blood pressure when taken daily. If you are taking cortisone by mouth or injections, it will temporarily raise your blood pressure. Some women develop hypertension when they take estrogen or oral contraceptives in any form.

Medicine for Lowering Blood Pressure

Twenty years ago doctors had only a few medications to lower blood pressure, and most of these caused side-effects. For this reason, patients fear blood pressure medicine. However, doctors now have numerous anti-hypertensive medicines with minimal side-effects. I will describe the types of medicines that lower blood pressure in more detail below.

Here is the new concept behind current blood pressure medicine. Blood pressure medicine affects the moment-to-moment tensions and chemical reactions in the walls of blood vessels that carry oxygen and nutrients. However, each drug by itself can correct only one problem. When only one drug is prescribed, the body often compensates by raising blood pressure to previous levels. A second medicine will block this compensatory response and may allow for lower doses of both medicines with fewer side-effects. A combination of more than one drug is often the best option, and these combinations are available in cost-saving single pills.

What to Look for in Research on Hypertension

Doctors suspect genetic variability in hypertension. Someday, when we understand more about the human genome, we will be able to test patients to see which medicine will work best. That will save time and expense, and prevent unnecessary side-effects.

Another promising area of research is based upon the fact that people have twenty-four hour timing surges in the level of their blood pressure. For example, the average person's pressure should be lower during sound sleep. However, some people have persistent elevations during sleep and, sure enough, this correlates with increased risk of heart attack and stroke. In the future, we may be recommending bedtime medicine to this subgroup to overcome this more dangerous variable.

Here is what I advise if you want to avoid the brain damage and dementia that could result from high blood pressure. Have your pressure checked at the doctor's office every year or buy a medium-priced blood pressure cuff for the upper arm (not the cheapest one, and not the most expensive one with all the bells and whistles). Check your blood pressure at home once a month. If your blood pressure is consistently higher than 130/80, you are at risk for complications. Your doctor will probably try weight loss and a change in diet first. If that is ineffective, and your doctor recommends medicine, make sure that you take it daily, keep getting follow-ups on your blood pressure, and be patient as your doctor adjusts the dosage and follows you for efficacy and side-effects.

The First Line of Defense:
Using Diet and Exercise to Prevent
Stroke and Protect Your Brain

The Simple Version

Daily aerobic exercise is the single most important thing you can do to prevent stroke. A blood pressure less than 130/80 and/or smoking cessation are also key to preventing stroke.

A twenty point drop in blood pressure can halve the risk of stroke or heart attack. A 20 lb. weight loss may drop the blood pressure 20 points, exercise may take 4 to 9 points off blood pressure, less alcohol may take off another 2 to 4 points, and a low salt diet may help lower blood pressure.

The Details

Before I tell you exactly how to protect your brain, I am going to ask you to ponder this philosophical issue. Life is about making choices, at least in a free country like the United States. You can choose to spend your money on cigarettes or medicine for lowering cholesterol or blood pressure. You can ignore your weight and eat fast food and sweets, and you can come up with any number of excuses to not exercise. Or you can choose to eat fresh fruits, vegetables and lean meat and make time for exercise in your daily routine. The choices you make now will greatly affect the health and integrity of your brain in the years to come.

I wish it were that simple. See the light and change your life. Regardless, people smoke and overeat to relieve stress. They forget to take their medicine, or they do not have enough money for it in a given month because the rent is a higher priority. They do not exercise enough because they believe they don't have the time. So, making the right choices now to preserve your brain will take effort. But the rewards to your health, emotions, peace of mind and overall mental clarity will be great.

When I tell you that you have choices, please understand that I am not judging older people who already have brain disease. Yes, maybe they could have made better choices but back when it might have made a difference to them, our present knowledge about how to preserve brain health was not available to them or to their doctors.

It is available to you. And that makes this generation very fortunate.

Exercise Helps to Prevent Stroke

Here is how exercise preserves brain function. Large blood vessels, which are analogous to interstate highways, deliver blood to the brain. More delicate vessels branch off from these large ones and carry the blood and oxygen to the remote areas of the brain, just as smaller roads carry supplies to little towns. Because the miracle of human brain function takes place when the connections between all the individual brain cells are working well, blood supply to every tiny area of the brain is important. If a single brain cell, loaded with intelligence, is cut off from the others, it cannot do anything for you.

When you exercise, the blood flow to these small vessels is increased. Exercise also stresses these delicate vessels in a controlled way when your pulse and blood pressure go up with exercise. By naturally stressing these tiny critical vessels with daily exercise, you are making them more compliant, more able to respond to a sudden surge in stress, adrenalin or a rise in blood pressure, such as when you are suddenly asked to speak in public or when you see the cop's flasher in your rearview mirror.

Physical inactivity raises the risk for hypertension and its associated diseases. Studies have shown that aerobic exercise (any activity that increases the pulse for a sustained twenty minutes or more) lowers blood pressure. Doctors also postulate that aerobic exercise lowers hypertension by reversing a condition referred to as Metabolic Syndrome (hypertension, abdominal obesity, diabetes, high insulin levels, low HDL).

Nutrition and Stroke

Can proper diet prevent stroke? Intuitively, we think that the answer must be yes, but proving that good nutrition keeps brain cells in better condition later in life would require serial brain biopsies, so "scientific proof" may be slow to materialize. Although our radiologists are becoming ever more sophisticated in brain imaging, the subtle changes that good diet makes would likely not be seen by serial scans over the years. One could certainly argue, however, that once there is any atherosclerotic plaque, we are already seeing the combined effect of genetic predisposition and a lifetime of poor diet and other lifestyle choices such as smoking.

In this case, we must employ common sense and the knowledge that we already have. Without a doubt, eating a good diet does have positive effects on your overall health. People need the antioxidants that are abundant in fresh fruits and vegetables. While oxygen is the very basic fuel of cell life, its by-products, called free radicals, may be toxic to cells. Anti-oxidants counteract free radicals.

Limiting salt to 2.4 grams (less than one and one half teaspoons) of sodium per day lowers blood pressure in some but not all patients. Doctors cannot yet predict which hypertensive patients will benefit most from a low salt diet. But ten years from now, as our knowledge of human genetics expands, we will be able to tell. The usual salt intake in the American diet is far above the recommended 3 grams. Most people ingest 7.6 to 10 grams of salt per day, (over 3 teaspoons). A lot of this salt is in processed foods; frozen dinners, canned goods, salty snack foods such as potato chips, nuts and pretzels, and restaurant or fast food. Only 20 to 30 percent of salt in the average diet is added at the table or used in food preparation at home.

Blood pressure can also be lowered by the potassium found in fresh fruits and vegetables, and the calcium found in dairy products or calcium supplements (1,500 mg. of calcium per day is recommended). The best diet for hypertension is called the DASH (Dietary Approaches to Stop Hypertension) diet. It contains all the elements listed above, along with menus, and is low in red meat and sweets, and high in whole grain products, fish, poultry and nuts. It has plenty of calcium, magnesium, potassium, and fiber. www.nhlbi.nih.gov/health/public/heart/hbp/dash/

Summary of Best Diet for Hypertension

Eat
- Fruits (but not as fruit juice)
- A rainbow assortment of vegetables
- Fish
- Poultry
- Nuts without salt

Avoid
- Pre-processed food
- Sweets, including sugary drinks
- Salt

Medicine to Prevent Stroke

The Simple Version

We've discussed what behaviors may help prevent brain cell death and stroke, but what about medicines? If your blood pressure is higher than 130/80 despite daily exercise and being at your proper weight, blood pressure lowering medicine will help you prevent stroke. Cholesterol lowering medications, the statins, have recently been shown to prevent stroke and probably also limit the plaques in the brain of Alzheimer's disease. Most doctors I know take a statin. Folic acid and fish oil will probably also preserve brain cells.

The Details

Although diet and exercise may normalize blood pressure, if you have a genetic predisposition to hypertension, you may need to do more. The blood vessels themselves have potent hormones, those little molecules that send messages from cell to cell and give operational commands. Hormones such as angiotensin and nitrous oxide influence blood vessel opening, closing, tension, and relaxation (compliance) to accommodate and direct blood flow. If you have inherited over-reactive blood vessels, you have to consider angiotensin converting enzyme (ACE) inhibitors. These are a class of medicines that dilate the blood vessels and turn off the constricting hormone in blood vessels, angiotensin. In the future, as a consequence of the decoding of the human genome, we may be able to tell early in life who has inherited stroke-inducing, overbearing angiotensin in his or her blood vessels.

One particular drug among the ACE inhibitors, ramipril (Altace) was shown to prevent stroke independently of its effect on blood pressure. Research over the next few years should tell us if this whole class of ACE inhibitor drugs has the same benefit. From my experience, I personally think all these drugs will help equally. Potential side-effects of ACE inhibitors are a dry cough, headache or, rarely, swelling of the lips or tongue called angioedema. If you can live with it, the cough is not sufficient reason to stop the medicine, but if you get the angioedema, you should not take this medication.

Some of my midlife patients are leery about taking blood pressure medicine.

When I suggest taking these medications to my male patients in their fifties, they pause, take it under consideration, then ask, "What does your husband, Mike, take?" I tell them that he has been on captopril 50 mg. twice daily since 1985 for hypertension. Both his parents had hypertension and he seems to have inherited it. He has tried other, newer, more expensive medicine, but none has worked so well for him with so few side-effects. Captopril has not "affected" Mike in any observable way. My patients are relieved to know that if my husband takes high blood pressure medicine, it probably won't hurt them and just might help.

The angiotensin-receptor blockers (ARBs) are a group of medicines that have an analogous effect on angiotensin but they take effect at a different place in the biochemical sequence. For this reason, they have fewer side-effects. The side-effects reported are palpitations and headaches. These newer ARB drugs are also more expensive. Other medicines may be necessary to achieve a steady state blood pressure below 130/80 and your doctor can help you to find the one that is right for you. Our current thinking, however, is that ACE inhibitors are the first choice.

The same drugs that lower cholesterol, HMG CoA reductase inhibitors or statins, such as Pravachol (pravastatin), Zocor (simstatin) and Lipitor (atorvastatin), also decrease inflammation in the blood vessels and lower C-reactive protein. I told you in a previous chapter that statins may limit the size and number of Alzheimer's amyloid plaques on the brain later in life. Now new research shows that taking statins may prevent a first stroke. But we are unsure whether this is accomplished by lowering cholesterol and decreasing inflammation, or through some other salutary effect on a person's blood vessels. Watch for new information about these medications in the near future. I expect to see studies of serial brain MRIs in people on HMG CoA reductase inhibitors compared with those on no cholesterol medicine. These studies should tell us whether or not taking statins prevents strokes.

Homocysteine is that amino acid that is potentially toxic to brain cells and blood vessels when it reaches a high level. Three B vitamins, folic acid, B6, and B12, lower homocysteine. If you have a homocysteine level over 15, doctors advise taking Foltx, Cerefolin, or Folgard, a prescription with these B vitamins in a single tablet. No proof yet exists that lower homocysteine prevents a heart attack or stroke, but we think that will be born out in future studies. If you take these vitamins individually, which would be cheaper, everyone should get at least 800 micrograms of folic acid daily. The recommended daily allowance of B12 and B6 is 2.5 mg. and 1 mg. a day respectively. We cannot be more precise than that in terms of body size, but the body will excrete any excess folic acid and B12 and it does not build up toxicity. There have been some cases of toxicity from those who took mega-doses of B6.

Fish oil may help to prevent stroke and dementia according to early studies that still need confirmation. Doctors regard it as a valuable and inexpensive adjunct to prevent and treat atherosclerosis, the underlying disease that causes stroke. Fish oil contains two different omega-3 (also called long-chain n-3) fatty acids: EPA and DHA. If your family does not eat two or three "oily fish" (tuna, mackerel, salmon, or sardines) meals a week, this supplement should be taken in combination capsules at a dose of 1000 mg. a day regardless of body size. The mechanisms by which omega-3 fatty acids slow atherosclerosis are several and complex. Fish oil probably works by decreasing inflammation in blood vessels and raises your HDL a few points. So far, no serious side-effects are known that require monitoring. Though there may be a slight fish taste an hour or two after taking the fish oil capsules, this can be eliminated by keeping them in the freezer and taking them at bedtime.

You may have heard about the threat of mercury in fish. Mercury does not tend to concentrate in the edible part of the fish that contains the EPA-DHA but rather in the liver. Therefore, cod liver oil is not a good choice. Mercury concentrations are most significant to women who are pregnant or of child-bearing age and to children since mercury can potentially be toxic to the brain of a fetus or young child. Most states have now made it a law to post notices warning of the mercury content in certain types of fish. According to the latest federal guidelines, the fish most likely to contain mercury are shark, swordfish, king mackerel and tilefish. On the other hand, salmon, canned light tuna, shrimp, pollock and catfish are low in mercury.

Aspirin also prevents stroke and sometimes one of the other more potent prescription blood thinners is necessary in a person who already has had a stroke. Most patients with atrial fibrillation take Coumadin (warfarin), a potent blood thinner that prevents these blood clots from forming and traveling to the brain. President Richard Nixon took warfarin for atrial fibrillation, but he died anyway in his eighties of a stroke from an embolus originating in his heart. Unfortunately, blood thinners are not 100 percent effective in preventing strokes, but they greatly decrease your risk of stroke.

What Do I Recommend to Prevent Stroke?

Most people will benefit from:

- One coated 81 mg. baby aspirin daily
- 800 micrograms of folic acid
- Blood pressure medicine if their blood pressure is consistently greater than 130/80
- Perhaps, a statin
- One gram of fish oil a day

Estrogen after Menopause: Recent Studies of Dementia and Stroke

Based on the findings of the Women's Health Initiative (WHI), women were told that hormone replacement therapy likely causes dementia and stroke if taken for more than 5 years after menopause. Do the underlying facts in those articles in medical journals support this notion? I will discuss WHI's claims about hormone therapy's effect on stroke and dementia separately.

The idea that hormones affect the brain is not a new notion. The brain is a sex organ; any woman who has been sexually active knows that. There are estrogen and testosterone receptors in the brain, particularly in the portion responsible for memory. Some evidence suggests that estrogen prevents the accumulation of amyloid plaques, the hallmark of Alzheimer's disease. Older studies show that women who take estrogen beginning at menopause are less likely to develop dementia.

However, the belief that estrogen could protect women's brains was questioned in the WHI. The website is www.NHLBI.NHI.GOV/whi, if you want to get to the source. The WHI Memory Study looked at 4532 women, aged 65 and older, and followed them for four years, testing them with a simple questionnaire, the modified Mini-mental Status Exam. Please note that the women studied were about 15 years past the average age of menopause. During the four years the WHI studied these women, a total of 61 women were diagnosed with dementia. The breakdown is as follows:

- 40 of the 2229 women assigned to the hormone group got dementia.
- 21 of the 2303 who did not take hormone therapy got dementia.
- The number of women diagnosed with dementia in both groups was actually smaller than would have been expected had nothing been done to these women or had they never been studied.

Based on the WHI study, the media and the scientific journals have been reporting that estrogen replacement therapy does not protect a woman's brain against dementia. However, this conclusion is problematic because of how the study was designed. It asked the question, "Does estrogen prevent dementia?" But to really discover the answer to this question, you would have to start treatment at menopause in women who had no dementia. The WHI study was done on women at the average age of 65. At that age, statistically, some of the women had to already have dementia.

The study was not designed to see if estrogen treated established dementia. Because the average age of the women in the study was 65, and they had never taken estrogen before, the question remains as to whether estrogen taken immediately after menopause could preserve brain function. This is when the symptoms of sleeplessness, irritability, decreased memory, and hot flashes are present, all manifestations of less than perfect brain function.

The test of mental function, the modified Mini-mental Status Exam, used in the WHI Study for dementia is crude and useful only as a screening exam. The women who supposedly developed dementia during the study period could have had dementia before they ever started estrogen, and the dementia could have been discovered had they been tested with more detailed and reliable neuropsychological tests or PET scans before enrolling in the study. Other studies using PET scans show increased metabolism in the memory areas of the brains of women who take hormone replacement, which contradicts the reported findings from WHI.

The public is easily misled by statistics. If you look at the numbers, the chance of any woman becoming noticeably demented, whether or not she started on estrogen replacement therapy at age 65, was already small. What the media reported is that the chance of getting dementia if you are on hormones is doubled. A women who is not a medical professional will read this and naturally interpret her personal risk as being 1 in 2 if she continues to take estrogen. The real risk of dementia in the study was one in one hundred for women not on hormone replacement, and one in fifty for those taking the hormones.

This Study Also Leaves Us With a Number of Unanswered Questions:

Since the body becomes insensitive to some medicines when they are administered on a continuous basis, does the same daily dose of estrogen affect brain cells the way cyclical estrogen might? Cyclical estrogen means three weeks on and one week off, simulating the menstrual cycle from earlier years. The body becomes insensitive to some medicines when they are administered on a continuous basis.

Is there a genetic difference in women's brain response to estrogen? Perhaps estrogen preserves brain cells in only some women. The authors of WHI surmise that those who develop dementia while they are taking estrogen have had small strokes because some women have an increased risk of blood clotting with hormone replacement.

The WHI Study only looked at cognitive function in women age 65 and older. What if there is a specific time before age 65, right after menopause, during which brain cells can be preserved by estrogen therapy?

Suffice it to say there is more controversy here than hard science. Expect this line of inquiry – the relationships of sex hormones on the aging brain – to become an area in which major advances may come in the near future.

What Do the Recent Estrogen Studies Show About Stroke?

When birth control pills first became available in the 1960's, we saw an infrequent but alarming side-effect – blood clots and strokes. This was one of the first clues that the female hormone pills might predispose certain women to clotting.

Part of the WHI looked at 16,608 women aged 50 through 79 to see if they had a greater chance of developing stroke on hormone replacement therapy (HRT). The average age at the start of the study was 63.3 years, and three fourths of the women had never taken estrogen after menopause before this study.

The majority of the women were Caucasian. Half of the women took no hormones and half received a combination of estrogen and progesterone. Progesterone is the hormone released by the body during the second half of the menstrual cycle. Unless a woman has had a hysterectomy, progesterone must be taken with estrogen replacement to prevent uterine cancer. Out of 16,608 women, followed for an average of 5.6 years, 151 of the women taking hormone replacement (HRT) had a stroke and 107 of the women who were not taking HRT had a stroke. Close to 80 percent of the strokes among those on hormone replacement were small vessel strokes. March, 2004, the WHI stopped the estrogen only arm of the study because of similar findings…a slightly increased incidence of stroke in women taking the medicine vs. those on placebo.

The study reports that the risk of stroke in women taking hormone replacement is 1.31 times that of women not taking it. Some women interpret that as meaning that their chance of a stroke is 1 in 3 on HRT. In reality, their chance is less than 1 in 1,000, whether they take hormones or not.

Some risks for stroke are far stronger than estrogen replacement therapy. These other risk factors include:
- smoking
- hypertension

- heart disease
- high cholesterol
- inactivity
- obesity
- family history
- inflammation in the blood as measured by the highly sensitive C-reactive protein.

The WHI study was designed to ask the question, "Do estrogen and estrogen/progesterone taken as a combination prevent stroke?" Once again, the average age of the women involved in the study was 63 years old. By that age, many of these women would have already had a small stroke whether they knew it or not. These strokes would have been significant enough to show up on a brain MRI, but no MRIs were done on enrollees at the beginning of this study.

Nobody believes that estrogen treats stroke, but we still don't know if taking estrogen beginning at menopause prevents stroke.

These Are the Questions That Remain Unanswered by the WHI Study:
- Do we really know if a woman may have increased blood clotting due to estrogen replacement? In all fairness, although the answer may be "only a few," if you are the one who has the stroke, it is 100 percent for you.
- Does the overall benefit that estrogen started at menopause has on the brain outweigh the risk of stroke later on?

The data to answer these questions are simply not available.

Epilogue

How I Advised Charlie to Protect His Brain from Stroke and Dementia

Charlie and I met as doctor and patient. I could see immediately that, like many men, he overestimated the level of his health and underestimated his health risks. The first thing Charlie told me was that he felt fine and had only made the appointment at his wife's insistence. He reported that his father had hypertension. He also had a grandmother who had dementia by age 70.

Charlie had some lifestyle habits that were not in his best interest, including smoking. He enjoyed fixing up old houses and spent some of his spare time, not always sober, up on a ladder painting and doing repairs. He fell once and was unconscious for a few minutes from a concussion.

Charlie was twenty pounds overweight and his blood pressure was 150/100. His blood tests showed a total cholesterol of 250 and an HDL that was low at 35. I checked his homocysteine level and it was quite elevated at 18.9mg/dl. It should be less than 9.5 mg/dl.

I agreed with Charlie's wife that he was at serious risk of being disabled by brain disease in his sixties or early seventies. For this reason, I encouraged him to stop smoking and to decrease his alcohol intake to one or two drinks, twice a week, or to quit drinking altogether. I advised him to lose twenty pounds and referred him to a dietician for a low-salt, weight loss diet. As a start, I asked him to work up to thirty minutes of daily aerobic exercise, such as walking on a treadmill. Before he began, however, I administered a stress EKG to make sure he would not have a heart attack when he started an exercise program. For his exercise to be really beneficial for him, ideally Charlie needs to increase his workout to forty-five to sixty minutes a day of exercise. After explaining how head injuries contribute to dementia, I instructed him not to get on a ladder again unless a second person was standing at the bottom, holding the ladder. And he should never get on a ladder or in any other risky position after drinking alcohol.

Since Charlie's blood pressure was too high, I started him on Altace (ramipril), 2.5 mg. gradually increasing to 10 mg. to bring his blood pressure down to our goal of 130/80 or less. To lower his homocysteine I prescribed Foltx, 2.5 mg. daily.

When I checked his cholesterol two months later, he had not succeeded in losing weight or lowering his cholesterol, so I prescribed an additional medication, Pravachol (pravastatin), 40 mg. at bedtime, to lower his cholesterol and improve the function of the cells lining his blood vessels.

As of this writing, Charlie's overall health is improving and his risk factors have been reduced. If he continues to follow my recommendations, his best outcome will be never suffering from either dementia or stroke.

In Summary, Let Me Highlight a Few Things That You Can Do to Help Prevent Stroke and Dementia:

- Keep your blood pressure lower than 130/80.
- Keep your cholesterol under 200.
- Do daily aerobic exercise ideally for up to forty-five to sixty minutes.
- Eat a rainbow assortment of five to six fresh fruits and/or vegetables daily.
- Take folic acid, at least 800 micrograms a day.
- Take a one gram capsule of EPA-DHA fish oil a day or eat two to three meals with fatty fish weekly.
- Don't smoke.
- Take one coated baby aspirin a day.
- Take Advil or another anti-inflammatory medicine a few times weekly.

Websites of Interest

Neurosciences Institute of San Diego and Dr. Gerald Edelman
http://www.scripps.edu/nb/chair.html

The Nun Study
http://www.mc.uky.edu/nunnet/

The Grant Study and Dr. George Vaillant's work
http://www.radcliffe.edu/murray/data/ds/ds0290.htm

Baltimore Longitudinal Study of Aging
http://www.memorylossonline.com/glossary/blsa.html

Brain CAT
http://www.radiologyinfo.com/content/ct_of_the_head.htm

Brain MRI
http://www.nlm.nih.gov/medlineplus/ency/article/003791.htm

Stroke:
http://www.strokeassociation.org and
http://209.107.44.93/NationalStroke/HavingAStroke

DASH diet (best diet for hypertension)
http://www.nhlbi.nih.gov/health/public/heart/hbp/dash/

Women's Health Initiative
www.NHLBI.NHI.GOV/whi

Glossary

Alzheimer's - The brains of Alzheimer's patients show characteristic sticky microscopic plaques of amyloid, degenerated proteins, and tangles that once were effective paths of communication among brain cells. They also show a marked loss of brain cells. Unless a person has died and his or her brain has been examined under the microscope, you can only say someone has probable Alzheimer's.

Amyloid Plaques - One of the two brain abnormalities that define Alzheimer's disease. Amyloid plaques are a sticky buildup that accumulates on the outside of nerve cells or neurons.

Aneurysm - A blood vessel with a thin wall that may balloon and suddenly burst, causing blood to spill out onto adjacent brain cells, which disrupts their blood supply.

Angiotensin Converting Enzyme (ACE) Inhibitors - These are a class of medicines that dilate the blood vessels and turn off the constricting hormone angiotensin.

Angiotensin-receptor Blockers (ARBs) - Another class of medicines that dilate the blood vessels by turning off the constricting hormone angiotensin.

Anoxic Encephalopathy - Loss of brain cells due to sudden loss of blood for example the heart stopping.

Anti-inflammatory Drugs - In addition to plaques and tangles, the brains of Alzheimer's victims also show signs of inflammation, immune cells that attack brain cells. Studies have shown that anti-inflammatories block this reaction and therefore, may also help prevent dementia.

APOE - A genetic marker for a protein carrier of cholesterol that comes in three basic forms, APOE-2, -3 and -4. APOE-4 is the gene that is associated with the plaques and tangles of Alzheimer's. A person gets one APOE gene from each parent. Two sets of the APOE-4 gene significantly increase one's risk of developing Alzheimer's.

Apoptosis - "Suicide" of brain cells. All cells in the human body are programmed to die eventually. However, in some brain conditions called neurodegenerative diseases, brain cells start to kill themselves early.

Atherosclerosis – The progressive narrowing of blood vessels all over the body causing the build-up of cholesterol-laden plaque.

Atrial Fibrillation - An abnormal heart rhythm in a weak heart that causes blood stasis and clots in the heart chambers.

Brain Cells - These cells consist of a nerve body with a long extension called the axon, which carries information to other nerve cells.

Brain Reserve - A term that describes the redundancy of connections on the brain. This is one of the issues that scientists consider in the study of dementia and Alzheimer's.

Caspases - Proteins that cause brain cell death.

Carotid Arteries - Found in the front of the neck, these are two of the four main vessels that carry blood to the brain.

CAT (computerized axial tomography) Scan - This test uses x-rays to map densities of brain tissue. Various areas of the brain, normal brain tissue, and injured brain tissue all transmit x-rays differently.

The Circle of Willis - A circle of blood vessels at the base of the brain that connect the two carotid arteries and the two vertebral arteries. This circle allows blood flow from one vessel to augment the others. Atherosclerosis in the Circle of Willis that blocks this cross flow can increase one's vulnerability to dementia.

Coumadin (warfarin) - A potent blood thinner.

C-reactive Protein - If you have an elevated level of C-reactive protein, which is a marker of inflammation, you have a propensity to develop atherosclerosis

Dementia - This term refers not to what one sees physically in the brain, but what one sees clinically in the patient's behavior. It literally means "lost mind." Many causes, including the plaques and tangles of Alzheimer's and/or stroke, can lead to the loss of function that we label as dementia.

Density of Ideas - A term used by Dr. David Snowdon, the author of The Nun Study, to define how many ideas a person expresses for each ten written words. Density of ideas reflects the brain's ability to process language, remember, and integrate thoughts.

Developmental Selection - A theory championed by Dr. Gerald Edelman that describes how specialized groups of brain cells begin, from birth on, to build basic brain functions when stimulated by new experiences.

Ego Defenses - The unconscious strategies that we develop to protect ourselves against life's big and small miseries have a lot to do with our happiness as we age. These defenses determine how well we can bounce back from tragedy and how effectively we are able to process stress while minimizing anxiety.

Dr. Gerald Edelman - A Nobel Prize winning researcher who is head of the Neurosciences Institute in San Diego. He is the author of A Universe of Consciousness: How Matter Becomes Imagination, which is one of the best books I have ever encountered on the complexity, versatility, adaptability, and emotional richness of the human brain.

Emboli - The clots caused in the heart chambers by atrial fibrillation. If these clots move to the brain, they can cause a stroke.

Experiential Selection - Dr. Gerald Edelman's theory that describes how every thought and stimulus, from the time we are born, has an impact on the critical neuronal connections that make up the mind.

Fish Oils – Humans need two essential fatty acids to survive, omega-6 and omega-3, which are both found in fish, especially the cold water variety such as salmon, mackerel, halibut, and herring. Fish oil probably prevents stroke and dementia.

The Grant Study - A long-term study authored by Harvard psychiatrist Dr. George Vaillant that explores what factors lead to happiness, health, and clear mental function later in life, and what factors leave some people bereft, alone, and suffering from diminished mental capacity. This study has shed significant light on the emotional factors that can help people to maintain efficient brain function as they age.

Gray Matter - The outer coating of the brain that contains the nerve cells.

HDL (high-density lipoprotein) - Also known as the good type of cholesterol, HDL moves cholesterol out of the blood vessels and back to the liver where it can be removed from the body.

Hemorrhage - When a blood vessel ruptures (hemorrhages) in the brain, spilling blood onto adjacent brain cells and disrupting their blood supply and function, a stroke results.

Homocysteine - An amino acid, or building block of protein, that all animals produce naturally. A high homocysteine level predisposes a person to stroke because it is toxic to brain cells and blood vessels.

Hypertension (a.k.a. high blood pressure) - A condition of persistently high arterial blood pressure. In adults this is usually defined as a blood pressure reading greater than 130/80.

Ischemia - A term that means loss of blood supply.

LDL (low-density lipoprotein) - Also known as the bad type of cholesterol, LDL moves cholesterol from the liver to atherosclerotic deposits in blood vessels.

Mini-mental Status Exam - A series of questions commonly used by doctors and researchers to test for dementia. This test is considered to be only a screening device and is not helpful in distinguishing the fine points of brain deficiency.

Modified Mini-mental Status Exam - A series of 100 questions used most often in research to test for dementia. This test is also considered to be only a screening device.

Myelin - A white sheath (similar to insulation) that wraps around the extensions of nerve cells in the brain and accelerates cell to cell communication. One could say that myelin is as important to the speedy delivery of brain messages as Federal Express is to the mail.

Neuropsychological Testing - A more detailed form of adult intellectual testing than the Mini-mental Status Exam.

MRA (magnetic resonance angiography) - A test designed to look at blood vessels in the brain. Using this technology doctors can see narrowed blood vessels that could potentially lead to stroke.

MRI (magnetic resonance imaging) - A strong magnetic field that measures the response of each hydrogen atom in the body to the magnet. The intensity of the response of the hydrogen atoms in the brain during an MRI depends upon the water content of the brain tissue, which will vary with different brain structures and different injuries. Two areas of MRI research are functional and perfusion MRI. Functional MRI uses sophisticated software to show areas of the brain that are active while performing a mental task. Perfusion MRI can estimate blood flow to different brain regions.

Neurofibrillary Tangles - An accumulation of twisted protein fragments inside nerve cells. These tangles are one of the characteristic structural abnormalities found in the brains of patients with Alzheimer's disease.

Normopressure Hydrocephalus - In adults a fluid build-up causing pressure around the brain.

The Nun Study - Begun in 1991 by Dr. David Snowdon, this is one of the most famous long-term studies about factors that might cause – or delay – the onset of dementia in later life. The study derives its name from the 678 retired Catholic sisters, aged 75 to 102, with whom Snowdon chose to work – an ideal population because of the uniformity of their diet, medical care, and lifestyle.

Off-target Verbosity – A communication style where a person talks too much, does not listen, and drifts from topic to topic. This conversational style is attributed to loss of the brain's ability to inhibit a person from saying everything he or she thinks.

Personality Disorder - A way of dealing with the world and other people based on a predominance of immature, offensive ego defenses.

PET (positron emission tomography) Scan - This test is able to very accurately measure the metabolic activity in the brain.

Plavix - A potent blood thinner that inhibits platelets clumping together in blood cells.

Re-entry - Dr. Gerald Edelman's theory about how a mentally active person is able to reconstruct skills and memories.

Small Vessel Disease - A term used to describe multiple small strokes, particularly involving the long stranded connections between brain cells.

SPECT (single photon emission computed tomography) - A test that uses radionuclides (radioactive sugar) to show blood flow to the brain.

SSRIs - Anti-depressants most commonly in use.

Statins - Cholesterol medicine such as Pravachol or Zocor (pravastatin or simstatin), which appear to decrease the formation of Alzheimer's plaques and tangles.

Stroke - Brain cell death due to a sudden loss of blood flow to part of the brain, denying cells enough oxygen and nutrients.

Subdural Hematoma - A blood clot outside the brain that causes pressure on it.

Synapses - The connections between brain cells. Many chemicals called neurotransmitters, such as serotonin, norepinephrine, and dopamine, pass across these synapses, allowing brain cells to communicate with each other.

Three Phases of Intellectual Decline - Decline in thinking ability with age has been categorized into three phases:
- Age-associated memory impairment (AAMI), usually not a precursor to dementia
- Mild cognitive impairment (MCI), probably a precursor to dementia
- Dementia or probable Alzheimer's

TIA (transient ischemic attack) - A temporary blocked blood flow to a part of the brain causing a temporary neurologic deficiency that clears spontaneously when the blood flow is restored.

Thrombus -When the plaque that has built up on the inside of blood vessels ruptures, platelets rush to the site and clump up to stop bleeding, just as they would at the site of any small cut on the body. Because a blood vessel is such a small space, the clump of platelets blocks off the flow of blood, causing a thrombus.

Vasculitis - Disease that directly inflames the blood vessels and may cause stroke in some individuals.

Vertebral Arteries - Found inside the bone of the cervical spine at the back of the neck, these are two of the four main vessels that carry blood to the brain.

Vitamin B12 - A deficiency of this vitamin may cause dementia.

White Matter - The part of the brain that contains all the long brain connections, found just beneath the gray matter.

White Matter Disease - A condition where multiple small strokes have affected the connecting filaments coming off the brain cells.

Women's Health Initiative (WHI) - Several ongoing long-term studies on the effects of hormone replacement on women later in life.

Midlife Medicine Series

Qty	Title	Price
	The Other Midlife Crisis: Arthritis and All Those Aches and Pains By Michael R. Wilson, M.D. An experienced orthopedist tells in plain words the causes of midlife aches and pains, arthritis and injuries, what works and doesn't in treatment. ISBN 0-9742976-0-7	$21.95
	Dispatches from the Frontlines of Medicine: Your Husband's Health: Simplify Your Worry List By Kathleen W. Wilson, M.D. For the concerned wife. How to keep him alive, and secrets to the quality of life problems, weight gain, fatigue, depression and erectile dysfunction. ISBN 0-9742976-1-5	$14.95
	Dispatches from the Frontlines of Medicine: Health for Midlife Women: When You Think You Are Falling Apart By Kathleen W. Wilson, M.D. Readers are empowered by understanding their changing bodies. From cosmetic surgery to hormone therapy, concerns midlife women have, presented in a clear, interesting way. ISBN 0-9742976-2-3	$21.95
	Dispatches from the Frontlines of Medicine: Brain Maintenance: How to Prevent Stroke and Delay Dementia By Kathleen W. Wilson, M.D. In the last two years doctors have found out how to prevent most dementia. Brain Maintenance makes this crucial information available and easy to read. ISBN 0-9742976-4-X	$14.95
	Subtotal	
	Sales Tax (if applicable)	
	Shipping and Handling $5.00 ($2.00 for ea. additional) U.S. $16.00 International	
	TOTAL	

Quantity discounts available.
Shipping time is usually 3-5 business days.

Shipping Address

Name _____

Address _____

City_____ State_____ Zip Code_____

Country_____

Telephone_____ Fax_____

E-mail_____

Billing Address
(if different from shipping)

Name _____

Address _____

City_____ State_____ Zip Code_____

Country_____

Name as it appears on your credit card_____

Credit card#_____cid#_____

Must include billing address for credit card if different from shipping.

Order by phone, fax, mail or online:

Whiskey Hollow Press
P.O. Box 13752
New Orleans, LA 70185-3752
•
Toll Free (866) 329-5710
•
Fax (504) 861-1657
•
www.boomermedicine.com

Make checks payable to Whiskey Hollow Press.

Books by Whiskey Hollow Press:

The Other Midlife Crisis:
Arthritis and All Those Aches and Pains
By Michael R. Wilson, M.D., Orthopedic Surgeon

Dispatches From the Frontlines of Medicine:

Your Husband's Health:
Simplify Your Worry List
By Kathleen Wilson, M.D.

Health for Midlife Women:
When You Think You Are Falling Apart
By Kathleen Wilson, M.D.

Brain Maintenance
How to Prevent Stroke and Delay Dementia
By Kathleen Wilson, M.D.

Notes